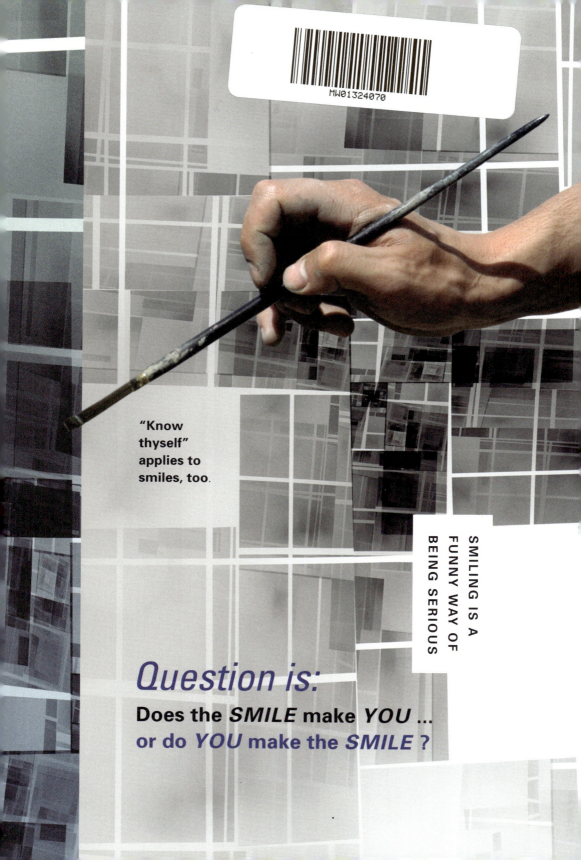

"Know thyself" applies to smiles, too.

SMILING IS A FUNNY WAY OF BEING SERIOUS

Question is:
Does the SMILE make YOU ...
or do YOU make the SMILE ?

your GUIDE TO THE PERFECT smile

What's in a smile?

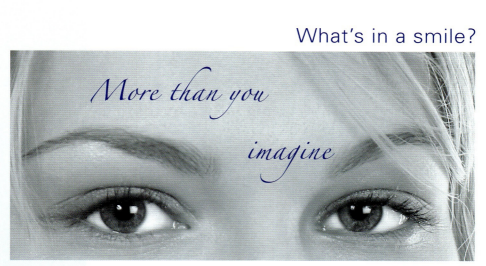

More than you imagine

EDWARD S. PHILIPS, D.D.S.

FOREWORD BY GERARD J. CHICHE, D.D.S.
AFTERWORD BY MARK BRESLIN

A BASTIAN BOOK

ECW PRESS
ecwpress.com

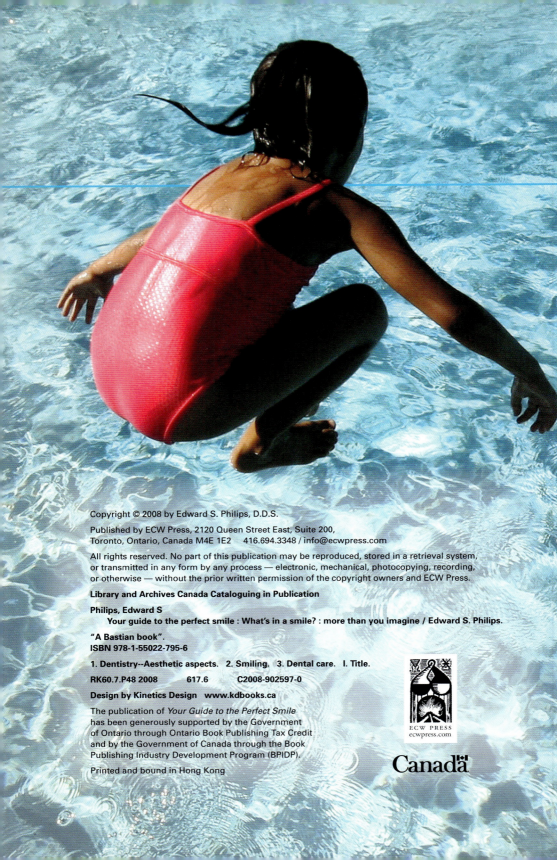

Copyright © 2008 by Edward S. Philips, D.D.S.

Published by ECW Press, 2120 Queen Street East, Suite 200,
Toronto, Ontario, Canada M4E 1E2   416.694.3348 / info@ecwpress.com

All rights reserved. No part of this publication may be reproduced, stored in a retrieval system, or transmitted in any form by any process — electronic, mechanical, photocopying, recording, or otherwise — without the prior written permission of the copyright owners and ECW Press.

Library and Archives Canada Cataloguing in Publication

Philips, Edward S
   Your guide to the perfect smile : What's in a smile? : more than you imagine / Edward S. Philips.

"A Bastian book".
ISBN 978-1-55022-795-6

1. Dentistry--Aesthetic aspects.   2. Smiling.   3. Dental care.   I. Title.

RK60.7.P48 2008   617.6   C2008-902597-0

Design by Kinetics Design   www.kdbooks.ca

The publication of *Your Guide to the Perfect Smile* has been generously supported by the Government of Ontario through Ontario Book Publishing Tax Credit and by the Government of Canada through the Book Publishing Industry Development Program (BPIDP).

Printed and bound in Hong Kong

Contents

Foreword v
by Gerard J. Chiche, D.D.S.

Preface ix

Introduction 1
"Give Me a Smile – a Perfect Smile"

1 **A Smile Comes to Dentistry** 9
Closing the Gap Between Dentists and the Public

2 **What's in a Smile** 27
Patterns, Stages, and Types

3 **The Big Picture** 43
Dentistry and the Aesthetic Principles of Nature

4 **Your Once and Future Smile** 57
Score Your Smile on the Ten Principles of Smile Design

5 **The Fix Is In** 77
Solving Common Smile Problems

6 **The Consultation Process** 113
Getting Comfortable with Your Dentist and Direction

7 **Before and After** 125
A Photo Gallery of Smiles

Afterword 137
by Mark Breslin

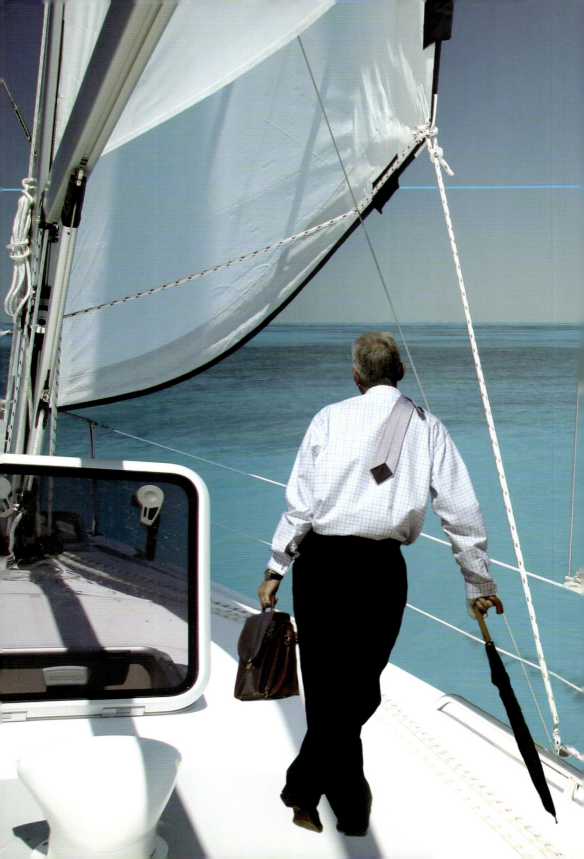

Foreword

I HAVE KNOWN ED PROFESSIONALLY FOR OVER FIFTEEN YEARS and am honored that he professes me to be his teacher and mentor. I do feel, however, that these accolades are unnecessary. After all, Ed, on his own merits, has pioneered advances in his own field of aesthetic dentistry. During our time as colleagues, I have enjoyed watching him develop the ideas of other colleagues and myself and rework them within his area of expertise.

My teaching and writing are focused on other dentists – and only indirectly on patients. Ed teaches dentists, too. However, he has always had a passion to "take it to the street." In this regard he has perfected what could be called a two-step translation process. First, he has taken his artistic and scientific understanding of the natural and aesthetic principles of beauty and put it into a technical, dental classification of the smile, with other dentists as his audience. Second, he has

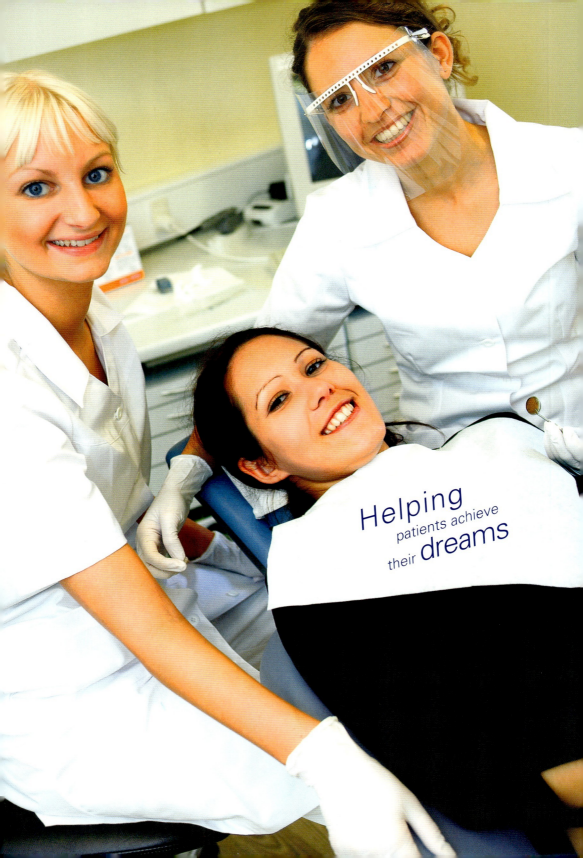

put this technical classification into a language that the public – the dentists' patients – can easily understand.

The effect of his efforts should not be underestimated. Dentists, dental technicians, and patients now have the ability to talk the same language as they work together on their dental realities and dental dreams.

The proof of Ed's prowess as a dentist and a communicator is in your hands. I am sure that this wonderfully entertaining and practical book will bring a smile to your face.

GERARD J. CHICHE, D.D.S.
Helmer Professor and Chairman
Department of Prosthodontics
School of Dentistry
Louisiana State University
in New Orleans

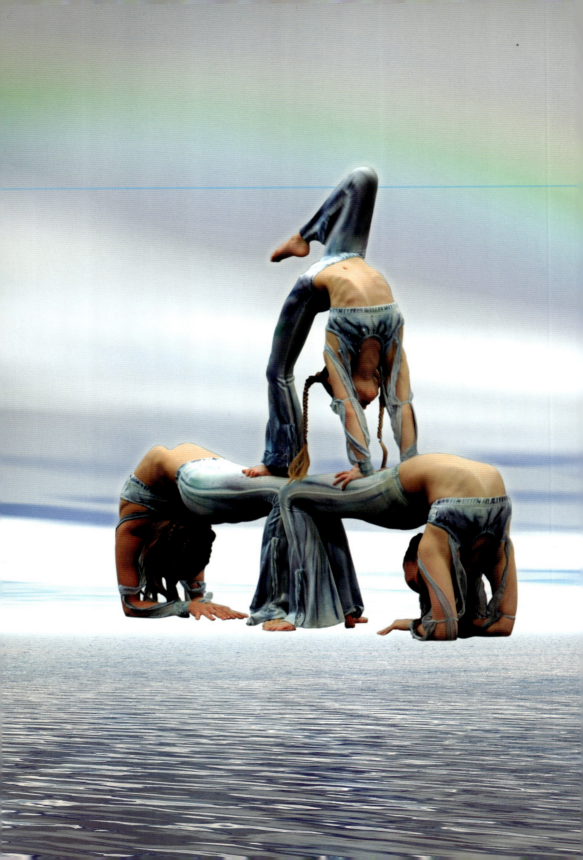

Preface

I HAVE MANAGED A SUCCESSFUL GENERAL DENTISTRY PRACTICE IN TORONTO SINCE 1979. However, in 1997 I decided to make a major change in how I practiced dentistry and in my lifestyle. Since that time I have concentrated my efforts on a separate and dedicated practice, the Studio for Aesthetic Dentistry. This practice, also in Toronto, is unusual, having only one chair, taking one case at a time, and focusing totally on dentistry to enhance people's smiles.

Through speaking, writing, research, and teaching, I have helped many dentists develop their understanding and practice of cosmetic dentistry. I have done this primarily through my definition of the smile and quantification of smile patterns, types, and stages, all of which are described in detail in this book.

I constructed my theories and methods out of necessity because I couldn't find courses, articles, books, or practitioners that gave me what I needed in a straightforward format.

I have written this book out of necessity, as well, in order to bridge a gap between patients and dentists. Numerous technical books are available on aspects related to the smile, but they are aimed at professionals and the public does not have easy access to them. Some general interest books on dental makeovers are out there, too, and they do give readers some details on the treatments that are available. However, they do not give them a language for expressing their subjective observations of their smiles such that their dentists can deal with those observations in a quantifiable, objective way. More specifically, till now, no book has been available to help patients and dentists score smiles on a methodical, ten-step system and put together a game plan for treatment.

...

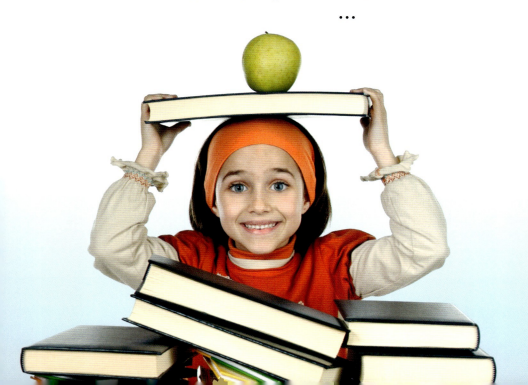

I owe a great deal of thanks to many people for their help in the development of the theories behind this book and for getting the book into your hands. Beyond my teachers, mentors, and my patients themselves, I want to thank my studio director, Billie Jo Sabo, who manages both my practice and me (the latter being her bigger challenge). As well, I would like to acknowledge my wonderfully supportive partners, Dr. Paul Custorei and Dr. Bob Feeley, who have stayed true to our partnership, giving me the freedom to explore my aesthetic needs at the Studio.

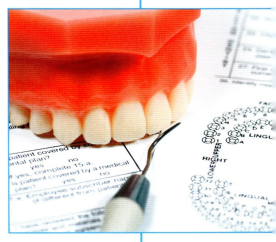

Till now, no book has helped patients and dentists put together a game plan for treament.

Of course, my greatest gratitude goes to my wife, Ann, and our six daughters: Yona (and her husband, Isser), Atara (and her husband, Dael), Adena, Shayna, Orlee, and Daniella. All have loved me, supported me, and cheered me on throughout the writing of this book, as well as throughout the years of discovery, study, and practice that preceded it.

Finally, I want to thank the power or powers that be for giving me a passion for life, a desire to grow and excel, to wake up every morning anticipating what the day will bring. Who knew?

EDWARD S. PHILIPS, D.D.S.

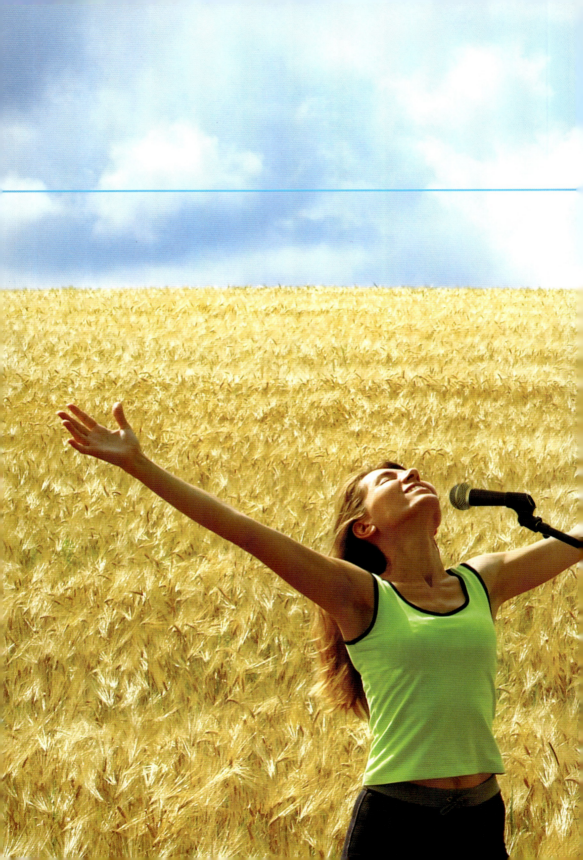

Introduction

"Give me a smile – a perfect smile"

In most cases, dentistry these days can comply with this request. The process, however, is not as simple as entering a hair salon and asking for a Jennifer Aniston or George Clooney look. It's true that a haircut is not just a haircut – to be good, it has to be right for the shape of the customer's head, face, and type of hair. But this is not even remotely comparable with the complexity of a smile's relationship to head, face, gums, teeth, jaws, distance between the pupils of the eyes – to mention just a few of the variables that come into play. The good news is that a transformed smile – transformed in a way that's right for you – will do more for your looks and self-esteem than any Hollywood haircut ever could.

As this book will show, the search for the perfect smile can be elusive, for you the patient and dentists alike. The complexities can hamper you in trying to state what you want and can stump dentists in delivering on your requests. Hence this book, the purpose of which is to help both patients and dentists communicate more clearly and effectively on their journey together.

The search for the perfect smile can be elusive.

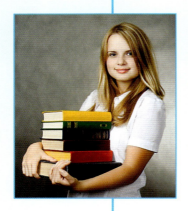

Giving you a basic understanding of how to achieve your desired smile.

If you are a patient, this book will help you by:

- Giving you a basic understanding of what's involved when dentists work with you to achieve your desired smile.

- Teaching you the language you need for discussing your wishes with your dentist.

If you are a dentist, it will help you by:

- Assisting you in interpreting your patients' requests. This is a complicated process. It involves sorting out perceptions, measuring desires against facial and dental realities, and turning their subjective needs into objective reality.

- Defining smiles for you, in terms of patterns, types, and stages, so that you can know how to get the right smile for the right person. *Your Guide to the Perfect Smile* also explores the techniques and processes that can be used in creating those smiles.

Things have changed a lot in society and in dentistry. What is motivating patients to undergo more comprehensive dental treatments these days is often not what's in their mouth but what's in their head. In traditional dentistry, patients had a tooth problem, and that's what they concentrated on. Relating to their dentist was very simple: "Here's my tooth problem," they could say. And dentists could say back to them: "Here's your tooth fix." Patients today, however, are often looking at their smile as one of several things to fix in a more complex set of needs –

whether to be more successful socially, express themselves more confidently at work, or just feel better about their image overall. With today's cosmetically conscious populace and in particular the Boomers aging energetically and youthfully and the strong social trend toward pursuing a healthy image, patients today are often approaching "Freedom 55" not as a retirement stage but a transitional stage. Putting their smile in check is just one of the tasks on their lists. They no longer have a tooth problem requiring a tooth fix; they have a head problem requiring a head fix.

Boomers are aging energetically and youthfully in the pursuit of a healthy image.

Before patients can feel that their dentist can fix their smile problem, they need to feel that their dentist cares about their head problem and can ensure that they will get the actual smile they are hoping for. This is so whether patients are looking for perfect pearly whites or a very natural but slightly worn look. In the face of these trends and patient desires, dentists should not try to be all things to all people. They may not be able to meet their patients' head needs on their own. Both dentists and patients need a dental team as a support system as they collaborate on an extensive smile fix.

In this book I attempt to capture the essence of my experience and teaching regarding smiles. In chapter one, I describe how the smile came to dentistry and the opportunities this has given dentists and their patients. In chapter two, I deal with smile patterns, stages, and types, and in chapters three and four with the aesthetic principles of nature and the principles of smile design. At that point, the question of how to actually create smiles based on this knowledge comes into play. Chapter five therefore examines specific smile problems and their solutions. Chapter six discusses what you need to know about the consultation process on your way to the perfect smile, and chapter seven closes the book with a photo gallery of before-and-after smiles and the stories that go with them.

It should be noted at the start of this book that the perfect smile you are searching for is not perfect in some ideal sense – it's the perfect smile for *you*. I have purposefully chosen pictures that are realistic, showing the beauty of a smile despite some deviations from the ideal. I've introduced a way of quantifying these imperfections, giving you the ability to score smiles, and have scored some of them myself in a section at the end of chapter four.

I've also made a conscious attempt to make the book entertaining. First, I have used artwork that goes beyond clinical photography to enhance the points I'm making. At times the message may be cryptic, so have some fun figuring it out. Second, I have included anecdotes called "Smilelines." These are meant to take you behind the scenes into the colorful world of aesthetic dentistry. You may want to skip these as you concentrate on the more factual information in the book. However, if that's what you decide to do, I hope you will come back and read them on their own.

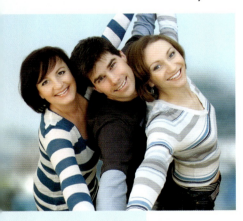

Your smile may already be perfect for you.

smileline #1

MY OWN VOYAGE INTO THE WORLD OF SMILES

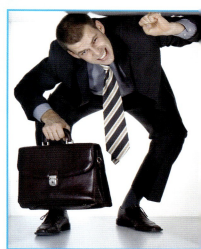

My main inspiration as a dentist and communicator has been Dr. Wesley J. Dunn, the dean of dentistry at the University of Western Ontario. His command of the language was awe-inspiring to me and other students. He was a man of tremendous presence. I was always nervous around him, prefacing every sentence with the words, "You know . . ." This infuriated him. I'll never forget how he once slammed his fist down on his desk and said, "If you say 'you know' one more time in my presence, I will throw you out of this office." I couldn't say a thing for the next forty minutes because, naturally, the loathsome words were now even more on the tip of my tongue.

Dr. Dunn had called me onto the carpet for being a little spotty, shall we say, in my studies.

"I don't understand you," he said. "This is the time when you should be showing brilliance, when you should be working really hard, and you're just sitting in your classes and acting as if it's not important."

His assessment of me – and it was accurate – was that I worked hard and did well when a course interested me, but was content to scrape by when it didn't.

Given my less than stellar performance, I was shocked when Dr. Dunn asked me – ordered me, really – to give a speech to dentists and professors of dentistry at the London District Dental Society meeting held during homecoming. Every year the school asked its leading students to put on such a presentation.

I had never made a speech in my life. Faced with this prospect, I did not want to be a leading student. I wanted to be a running student.

"Pick a topic like hypertension and dentistry," he said. "Don't worry. Giving a presentation is not hard."

It was hard. Really hard. But I did what he asked, to an audience of about 150 people, and it went over well. Dr. Dunn sent me a beautiful letter, saying something like, "Your knowledge belies your tender years."

I had never heard the word "belies" before and thought he was quoting an English poet.

The presentation helped me catch the eye of Dr. Gerald Z. Wright, head of the pediatric dentistry department. He enlisted me in breaking a barrier for UWO's dental faculty. No one from the program had ever landed an internship in a Toronto hospital. Though the dental school was coming on strong, and is now one of the best in Canada, at the time it was second tier.

Dr. Wright planned a pre-emptive assault on this barrier, and I was his cannon fodder.

"Come with me. We're going to Toronto," he said, hauling me off to the Hospital for Sick Children. We stormed – well, he stormed, anyway – into the office of Dr. Arlington Dungy, head of the dentistry department at the hospital.

"Dr. Dungy," he said, "this kid is good, good enough for an internship in your hospital. I've taken the time out to come down here with him to ask you to cut through all the bureaucracy and let him in. Dr. Dunn and I want this kid to work at Sick Kids to show you what we're teaching our students."

I was hired, and my internship in the dentistry department at Sick Kids, in 1978 and 1979, would prove foundational to my later work in cosmetic dentistry and my understanding of the smile.

I was assigned to work with the cranio-facial department on controversial, advanced work, along with plastic surgeons; speech pathologists; oral surgeons; ear, nose, and throat doctors; neurosurgeons; and social workers. The leading surgeon was Dr. Ian Munroe, a world-renowned cranio-facial surgeon now practicing in Texas.

Surgery in this department involved taking apart

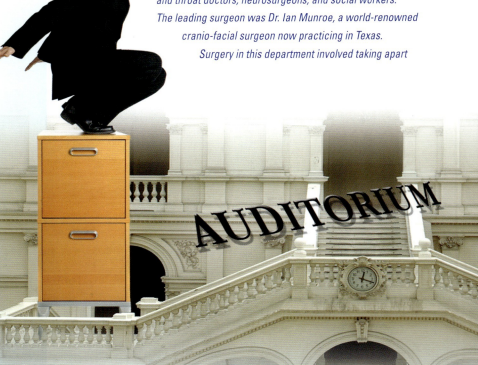

and putting back together again the faces of kids with major congenital abnormalities. As part of this process, the surgeons would move the jaws forward or back and needed a dentist to wire the jaws into their new position. Once the jaws were fixed, they could start to put the facial bones back where they wanted them. I went from learning the simple process of filling a cavity in a tooth to helping with total face reconstructions alongside experienced professionals from various medical specialties.

The experience was an object lesson for me in the fact that dentistry involves far more than teeth. The surgeons asked me questions that went way beyond what was being taught in dentistry and way beyond anything I could find in dentistry books and journals. I often had to admit I didn't know what to do and then figure things out the best I could.

After that year, I went on to work in general dentistry. After five or six years, however, I became restless. The work I was most interested in did not fit general practice. I attended lectures and conducted research that went beyond regular dentistry and into surgical and cosmetic issues. I was lucky to have as a mentor Dr. Gerard J. Chiche, chairman of prosthodontics in the School of Dentistry, Louisiana State University in New Orleans. I attended his seminars whenever possible and studied privately with him as well.

In the late 1990s, while continuing my business involvement in the general practice, I established a practice devoted solely to cosmetic dentistry. During the ten years since, I have also taught a great many dentists in Canada, the United States, and abroad, sharing my experiences and insights.

Most of the principles I've come up with were influenced, one way or the other, by teaching and research within the various disciplines of dentistry. However, I had to conduct research in other fields, notably plastic surgery, to complete my methodology. I am not the sole inventor of my definition of the smile or my "atlas" of smile patterns, types, and stages. Rather, I have taken points and insights that I saw here or there and worked and reworked them into a methodology with explanatory and clinical strength.

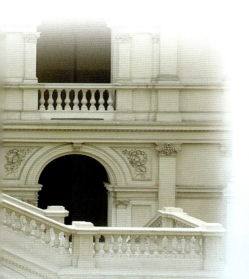

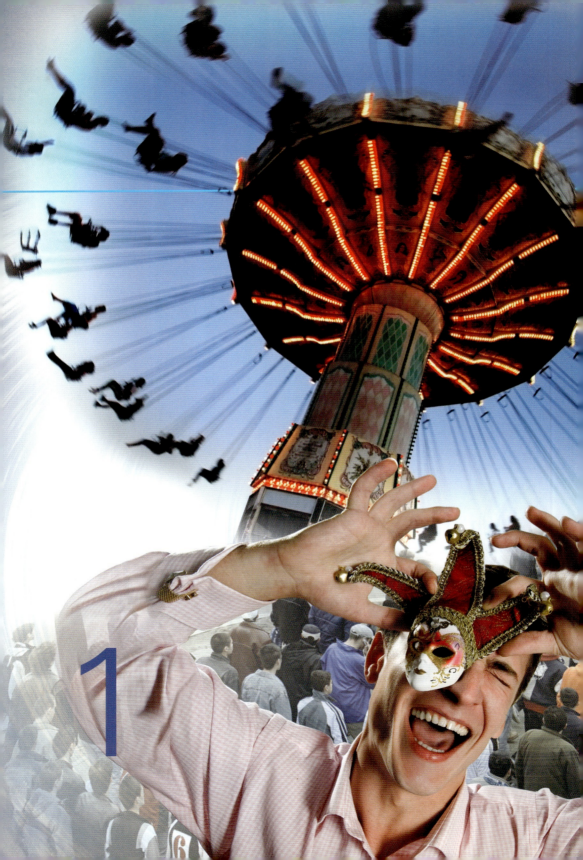

A *Smile* Comes to Dentistry

Closing the Gap Between Dentists and the Public

Until recently, dentists concentrated on straightforward, easily definable tasks. Cavities were filled. Toothaches were treated. Stained teeth were cleaned up. Hopeless teeth were extracted. Crowded teeth were straightened.

Over time, dental patients learned how to identify and communicate their needs and had a good idea of what dentists could do to meet those needs. Things are different now. Waves of plastic surgery, makeovers, and the desire for eternal youth have delivered a different kind of patient onto the shores of dentistry. These patients are asking for a lot more than dental care. They want dental beauty. They want a perfect smile.

In contrast to their cavity-filling years, however, patients today do not know how to express their needs and desires. They do not know what procedures are available. They're not even sure that their family dentist is up to performing the new procedures they're hearing and

Patients are asking for a lot more than dental care. They want dental beauty.

reading about. They worry that their dentist will be offended if they ask for a referral.

In the aesthetic world outside dentistry – such as plastic surgery – it's quite acceptable for people to leave their doctor and seek expert help themselves. They do not have to have a prior relationship with that expert. In the world of dentistry, however, you can't just go to another dentist, because that would require dental records to be changed.

Seeking an elective dental procedure is therefore quite difficult for members of the public. How do you get a second opinion without upsetting the dentist you may have no problem with?

Moving beyond different types of holes in teeth and different ways to fix them.

Many dentists are confused, too. They may have the technical skills to perform the underlying procedures that will result in improved smiles, but they often do not know how to analyze and quantify *actual* smiles, much less *desired* ones. It's easier for a dentist to deal with a smile problem when the person's teeth are in bad shape. The problem comes when when a patient's smile problem is not that serious. In that case, there is a danger that the patient – and the dentist – will be surprised by the results of the procedure, with the patient saying, "That's not what I wanted at all."

Fortunately, for everyone, most dentists know not

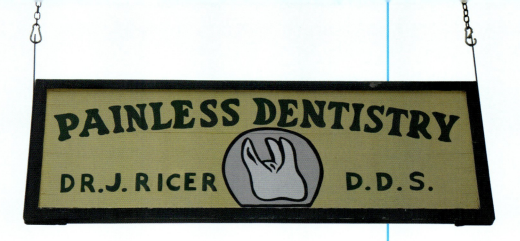

to get involved if they cannot understand a request or come up with a clear solution to a request.

The Evolution of Dentistry

Today's gap between patients and dentists can be traced in part to the evolution of dentistry itself. Only one hundred years ago, dentists were right in there with barbers and blacksmiths in terms of their development. Dentists lacked definitions or understanding of processes. They were operating by the seat of their pants.

Within those ten decades, however, dentistry moved light years ahead. All scientists and scientific practitioners depend on their ability to define the unexplained, and dentistry proved to excel in this ability. As the profession developed, dentists began to learn that there were different types of holes in teeth and different ways to fix them. That was good because patients began to get used to different types of problems and the solutions available for them.

Not only did this give patients comfort, but it also gave dentists as a professional body ways to confer on problems and solutions. Being able to agree that a certain type of cavity was class 1 or class 2, and so on, allowed them to come up with more nuanced diagnoses and treatments.

So, as a result, cavities became classified and dentists were able to develop better ways to treat patients and speak to them about the pros and cons and limitations of any treatment.

Periodontal surgery had a similar development. After a while, periodontists, who deal with gum disease, realized

Dentists were right in there with barbers and blacksmiths in terms of their development.

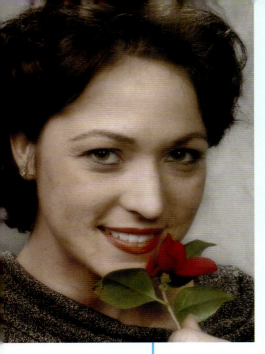

Who was fixing smiles?

that there were different levels and stages of this disease. Again, class 1 and class 2 designations, for example, were developed to help these dentists develop their ideas and treatments and to help patients understand the diagnosis and treatment of their problem.

The same was true of orthodontists. Their craft was to straighten teeth, but there was crooked and there was *crooked*. They needed language to say to a patient, "You've got an overbite, underbite, or crossbite." So names were given for occlusions: class 1, class 2, and class 3. Orthodontists went on to develop subdivisions within these classes.

But the challenge of definition was greater in the newest area of dentistry, smile dentistry. It was extremely difficult for dentists to discuss these problems and solutions with patients or other dentists. For a while, the health of the teeth, not the health of the smiles, was being analyzed. There was no definition of the smile that took the underlying reality of smiles – the rest of the face – into account. Patients could leave a dental examination knowing they had healthy teeth. But as for whether they had a healthy smile – both they and their dentists were at a loss. If you had asked patients, "Did your dentist check your smile?" the answer probably would have been, "I don't know. I'm not really sure."

The most fundamental question was, who was fixing smiles? The cosmetic companies claimed some responsibility, with their lipstick advertisements showing women with gorgeous smiles. Plastic surgeons were beginning to beautify lips by making them thicker, but they didn't really fix smiles unless they were dealing with patients who had been in car accidents or needed a surgical procedure.

So patients turned most often to their dentists. And dentists, true to their solid history in this regard, began to think through what they needed to do to fix smiles. To that point they were treating all smiles as essentially the same. They were fixing teeth. They hoped that great teeth would automatically result in great smiles. But I quickly realized that people don't all smile the same way and therefore that fixing patients' teeth the same way would not necessarily result in good smiles for them.

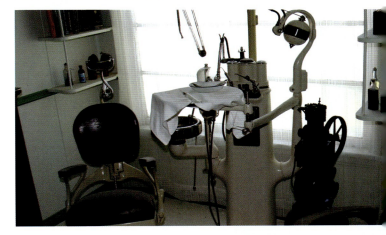

Healthy teeth did not necessarily mean a healthy smile.

The smile would not really come to dentistry, however, until certain demographic and economic realities played themselves out.

In the decade and a half following World War II, a lot of people did not have healthy teeth. They spent a great deal of time in the dentist's chair getting their teeth filled. By the time they were adults, many of them had almost as much metal in their mouths as teeth.

In the late 1950s and early 1960s, the lexicon of dental

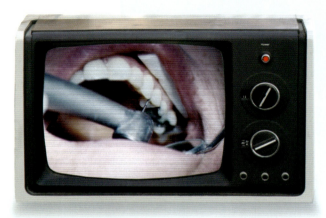

treatment sounded like an armed forces manual. Terms like armamentarium, high-speed drills, high-volume evacuation, extension for prevention, and four-handed dentistry were common. The mouth was a combat zone as dentists waged an all-out war against cavities.

The mouth was a combat zone as dentists waged an all-out war against cavities.

If that was the ground war, the air war consisted of two campaigns. In the first one, cavity-preventing fluoride was added to community water supplies. By the 1960s, this meant that, for the first time ever, children had naturally good teeth – they didn't require anywhere close to the number of fillings as the previous generation. In the second campaign, dental plan coverage was introduced, ensuring more regular visits by patients who were now less afraid of dental bills.

By the 1970s, dentistry was able to move from combat to peacekeeping. Prevention became the name of the game, as patients took advantage of new technologies. Increased insurance meant more regular check-ups – and topical fluoridation in toothpaste and after cleanings meant there were fewer problems. Besides fluoride, new dental procedures and technologies that were dominant in this period included periodontal therapy, pit and fissure sealants, and chlorhexidine rinses.

Then, in the 1980s, came the greening of dentistry.

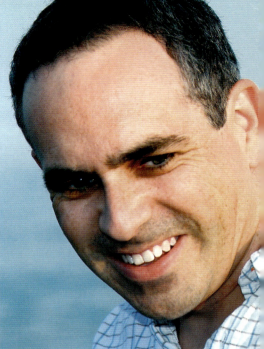

Dentists moved out of peacekeeping and into the recycling business. Patients who had sustained the crude, mechanical treatments of the 1950s and 1960s were forced by the deterioration or outdatedness of that work to return to their dentists for reconstructive treatments.

The generation that first benefited from prevention – let's call them the Flower Power generation of the 1970s and on into the 1980s – needed less care but expected more than baseline dental health. They wanted dental beauty. Or at least their parents wanted it for them. Remember the number of kids during those times whose smiles were bristling with wire braces?

Enter the generation of the decades straddling the turn of the millennium. These patients, and their dentists, now had the desire, time, ability, and technology to focus on the next level of care: the smile.

And that is how the smile came to dentistry. Today, all patients are concerned about the effects on their teeth of aging: their teeth are wearing down, their gums are receding, and their teeth are discolored. Some are consulting dentists about their smiles in connection with the plastic surgery they are anticipating.

Today's patient needs less care and puts a higher value on aesthetics.

Defining the Smile

There was something a little crazy about all this for me and many other practitioners in the 1990s when the most recent demographic wave got rolling. Patients were asking for their smiles to be fixed. New technologies were available to help make that happen. But, maddeningly, dentists weren't able to quantify what patients were requesting. How big? How small? How natural?

When I was planning to open a practice devoted to smile dentistry, I began to think about the public and the dental profession's need for definitions. It was only natural for me to look for these definitions in the literature of dentistry. But I was surprised by how little I could find there. I also looked into the theory and practice of plastic surgery and was equally surprised that many such surgeons were fixing smiles with no thought to the realities of the underlying teeth.

It seemed as if I was starting from the very beginning.

It seemed as if I was starting from the very beginning. I even had to look up "smile" in my trusty Webster's dictionary:

smile 1. *n* (Change of) facial expression, usu. with parting of lips and upward turning of their ends, expressing amusement, pleasure, affection, skepticism, contempt, etc.; (fig) pleasant or encouraging appearance. **2.** *v.i. & t.* make or have a smile (come up smiling, colloq., recover from adversity and face future optimistically); look pleasantly, encouragingly, propitiously, or scornfully (*at, on*, etc.; lit. or fig.); express by smiling (*smiled* a welcome, *smiled* her appreciation); give (smile) of specific kind.

What a strange situation: Dentists were increasingly considered to be in the smile business, yet the actual definition of the smile didn't even use the word "teeth." I remember wondering about myself and my fellow dentists, "So how, then, are we going to change their smiles? Are we planning to become psychiatrists?"

Eventually I came up with my own definition by adding to the dictionary definition the words:

> ... and the manner in which facial muscles, lips, gingiva, and teeth blend to create a pleasing expression.

This only made sense because the work dentists do on teeth affects the facial muscles. If we change the way someone bites, either by moving the jaw forward or back, this changes the hard tissue, which affects the soft tissue. If you change the underlying teeth or bone or jaw, you affect the face and hence the smile.

My definition therefore brings into focus what dentists do when it comes to fixing smiles. Our work affects the lips. By lengthening teeth, for instance, we make the upper lip thicker. By changing the arc of the shape of the teeth, we change the way the curve in the lips can go out. We can fix smiles that are too gummy by cutting the gums back or by moving the jaw up.

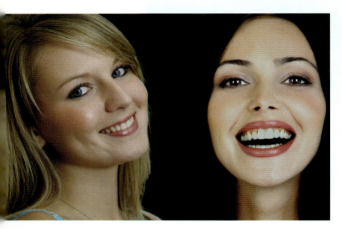

I made it my mission to quantify the smile by defining the smile scientifically. Out of this work, I developed the terminology of smile patterns, types, and stages, all of which will be discussed in greater detail in chapter two.

Aesthetic vs. Cosmetic Dentistry

Aesthetic dentistry and cosmetic dentistry have quite different purposes.

Many in the public – and in the dental profession – were also confused regarding the terms "aesthetic dentistry" and "cosmetic dentistry." In attempting to bring some clarity to this, I defined aesthetic dentistry as "a rehabilitative procedure to correct a functional problem using techniques that will be least apparent to the remaining natural peridontium and/or associated tissues."

Aesthetic dentistry is supposed to be transparent. It is beautiful, pleasing dentistry. Its results don't look artificial. The teeth are left looking natural. This is an exaggeration, but if someone whose teeth were completely black broke a tooth, aesthetic dentistry would fix the tooth and make it black to blend in naturally. Cosmetic dentistry, in contrast, can be seen as "an elective procedure to alter the existing natural or unnatural peridontium and/or associated tissues to a different set of values that the patient perceives will enhance their appearance." So in the case of the person with black teeth, the solution would be to fix that one tooth and make all of the other teeth white. Today, such a person is more likely to say, "I broke my tooth but I've always hated my black teeth. Can you fix them all?"

The Smile in History

Some people mock those in search of a perfect smile. They regard them as being on a vain exploration for the fountain of youth. These practical types see their dentists as mouth mechanics to be visited for regular check-ups and repairs. As far as they are concerned, asking their dentists for a better smile would be like asking their mechanics to make their sagging vehicles as good as new.

Some patients who seek the help of dentists seem to be aware of this perception. They are almost apologetic when broaching the subject of fixing their smiles. I have always assured them that they are not asking for something frivolous.

Far from it. I became more and more certain of the importance of smiles as I researched the scientific, anthropological, and historical literature. I found that the smile is a universal reality across all time periods and races. It is a primary expression from birth. The "use" of smiles varies from culture to culture, but if people from various countries were shown a photograph of a happy, smiling face, they would almost all agree on their interpretation of it. They would also concur in their interpretations of expressions of disgust, surprise, sadness, anger, fear, and contempt. Beneath all the complexity of humankind lies

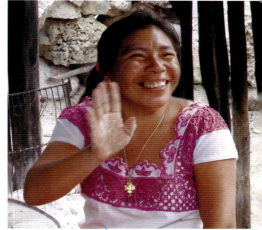

The smile is a universal reality across all time periods and races.

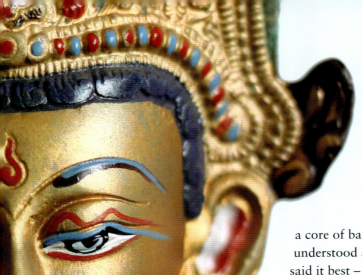

a core of basic emotional expression understood all over the world. Darwin said it best – that we all smile in the same language.

We all smile in the same language.

I researched the smile through the lens of evolution. It was clear that the main weapons in the arsenal of humankind in primate form were the hands and the mouth. Those with the most powerful jaws were at the top of the heap, because the more powerful the jaws, the better the hunting – and the control of one's peers. Territorial dominance was best achieved by the exposure of a powerful snarl. Not surprisingly, the jaws of early humans were much larger than ours today. The smile would be seen with gaps, sharp, uneven incisors, and large, over-erupted canines. The purpose of jaws and teeth was not only to serve as powerful weapons but also to help their owners chew foods that were tough in their raw, uncooked state.

As the human race developed, physical and sociological needs changed. We continued to have the same genetic response to strength and authority. But now our focus on the jaws accorded primacy to those whose smiles were naturally, architecturally balanced in a flowing, curved

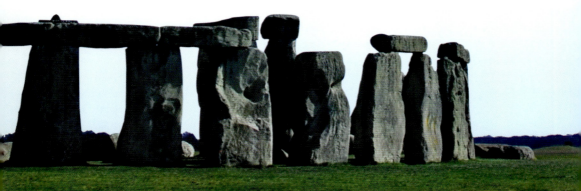

face. Gone was the need for a large jaw and fearsome teeth. We weren't looking for proof of aggressive power but for a feeling of community. This was a radical change. Where teeth were once used to keep people away, their function now was to attract them. The same genetic programming was in place. Our eye is genetically programmed to focus on the mouth for sociological cues. However, now the smile is seen to convey compassion, understanding, enjoyment, and affirmation.

Physiologists and psychologists agree that neurological aspects of the smile have psychological effects. People with strong, pleasing smiles are more successful in business. They do better in school. They do better in romance. Psychologist Robert Zajonc postulates that when a person smiles deliberately – even when feeling blue – the brain releases neurotransmitters that can override their sadness. Studies by the psychologist Paul Ekman support this by showing the neurotransmitter effects of smiling. People who are sad or depressed feel better if they force themselves to smile. According to Jane Lyle, author of the book *Body Language*, many experts believe that smiling and laughing are beneficial to people's health. Ekman supports this theory, showing that even when unhappy people feign a smile, their heart rates slow down and their bodies become calmer.

Far from being vain or egocentric, people who contact their dentists for help with their smiles are being quite rational. In fact, as we will see in the following chapters, they are acknowledging the importance of design and aesthetic harmony in our perceptions of nature and art.

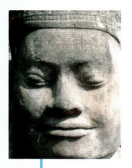
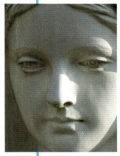
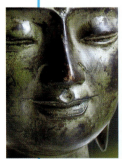

The function of smiles was now to attract people.

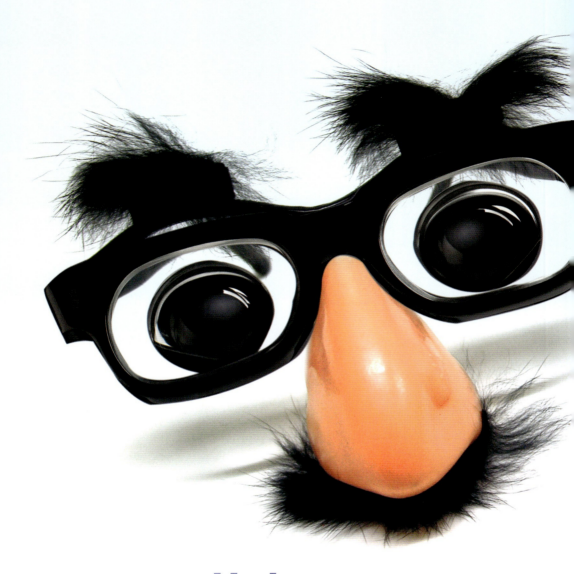

smileline #2

GETTING A BETTER LOOK

It's amazing what a few years of experience can do to change your perspective.

I was very excited when I got my first chance to do some actual clinical work during my training at dentistry school. It was around 1975. My assignment was to take a mold of someone's teeth and make a crown for a tooth.

This was my big day, the day I was to show my assignment to the professor in charge of inspecting our workmanship, the day my brilliance as a student was sure to be recognized and entered into the annals of my school.

When I met the professor I was even more excited. Here was an older gentleman with curly white hair who looked like a more academic brother of Santa Claus. Surely I was going to pass this assignment with flying colors.

After the briefest of greetings, he took my mold and looked at it closely. He didn't seem the least bit impressed. I started to squirm when his lack of adulation turned into a look of concern.

"Let me take a closer look," he said. Then he did something I had never encountered in my training: He flipped magnifying loops over his already thick glasses. Santa's brother had morphed into Groucho Marx with a thyroid problem.

"This is absolutely unacceptable," he grumbled a few moments later. "You are going to have to redo this completely" – whereupon he gave me some very specific instructions. I couldn't accept his assessment. I was so frustrated. I remember complaining about the situation to my long-suffering fellow students. "Here I am, a young guy with great eyesight, and who do they give me to but an old guy who can't even see properly."

Later I realized what an inspiring teacher he was. At that time it was rare for dentists to work with magnification. I was too unpolished to realize that this old guy was ahead of his time, a very skilled dentist teaching kids great work.

Today, magnification is routinely used by dentists. The principle is that the greater the magnification, the better your dentistry will be. The tradeoff, however, is that the greater the magnification,

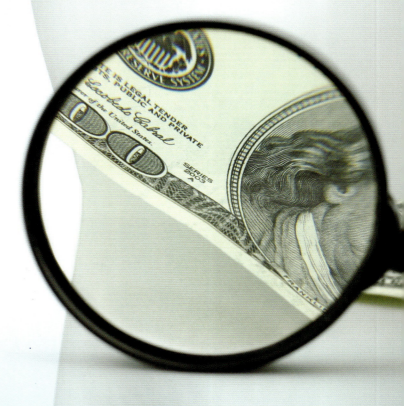

the harder it is to actually do the work. Why? Because you see more and you see less. You see more of what you're working on and your hand movements have to be that much more precise. But you see less – less of the field, of the area around the part you're working on.

All this means that the dentist with more magnification is not necessarily a better dentist. The challenge is for the dentist to get the right amount of magnification for their hands and eyes to have the right amount of control, while not losing a sense of the field.

Today, 4.5 magnification is considered strong but usable. And some dentists work with microscopes. They're not actually looking in the patient's mouth directly. Their hands are in the patient's mouth, but they are watching a monitor.

Today's dentists who have mastered the art of working with magnification are able to do particularly precise and beautiful work in such procedures as adding porcelain veneers, doing microsurgery on gum lines, and even performing deep root canal surgery.

Does magnification make you see *more* or *less*?

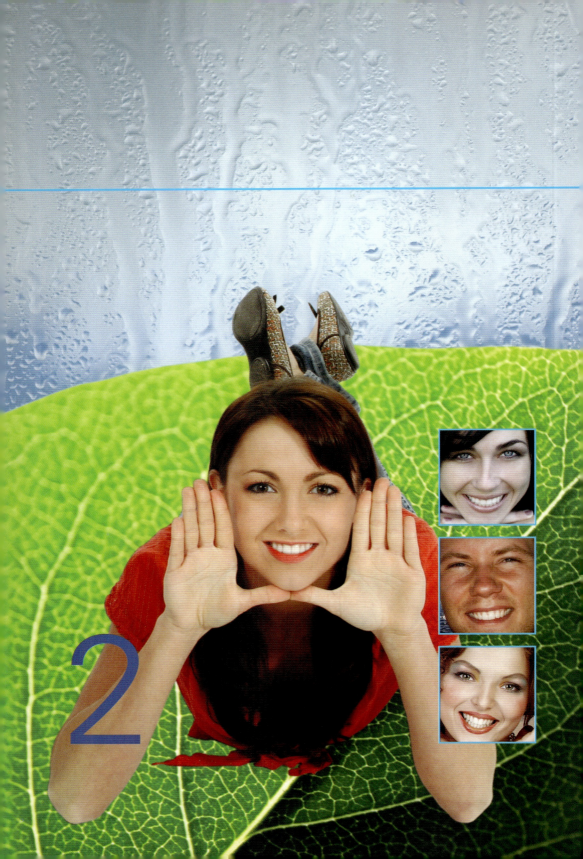

What's in a Smile

Patterns, Stages, and Types

KNOWING YOURSELF IS OF PARAMOUNT IMPORTANCE IN ANY AREA OF YOUR LIFE. That's the message of today's Tony Robbins as he inspires Fortune 500 executives to believe in the power of self-knowledge. It was the message in ancient times, too, when the Greek philosopher Socrates said, "Know thyself." Self-knowledge comes into particular focus when you're thinking about having work done on your smile.

People often come to me with a picture of Julia Roberts or Pamela Anderson and say, "I want that smile." If I tell them it's not possible, they panic. They think there's some kind of shortcoming in their treatment or that they have a problem that can't be fixed. I quickly explain that the challenge is not for them to get a specific smile they like, but to get a smile that likes them – one that is right for them.

Think of it this way: The most efficient way to shop for shoes is to ask to see everything the store has in your size.

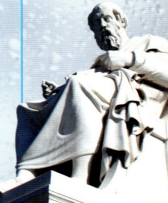

"Know thyself" applies to smiles, too.

There's no point in lusting after shoes that are too small or too large to begin with. The perfect smile for you is one that fits you, one that's in harmony with your facial realm.

The beginning of finding your perfect smile is for you to find out who you are. If you and your dentist can work together to understand the way your muscles, face, and jaws all work and to identify your smile pattern, you can get your perfect smile. The dentist must match the angles, the lines, and the emergent form of your face, teeth, and smile. If they can get your teeth to follow your face lines properly, then you will actually have the right smile for you.

To understand this better, think about lipstick companies and their advertisements. They show the different ways that different lipsticks affect the lips, and vice versa. They show lips that are round, oval, ovoid, long, thin. They illustrate how different colors of lipstick enhance certain aspects of the look of the person. In the same way, dentists, even though they may not fully change your smile, can enhance aspects of your smile by understanding your current smile, your desired smile, and the many variables of your facial structure, jaws, and teeth.

Different colors of lipstick enhance certain aspects of a person's look.

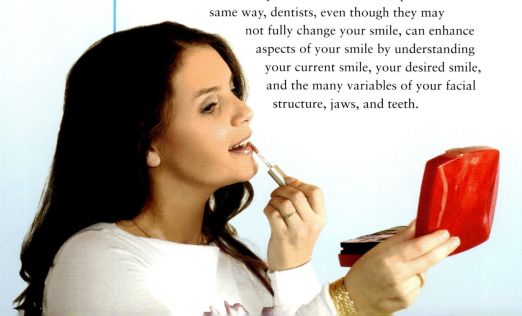

The Search for a Classification of Smiles

Not that long ago, to do the above was a major, and in most cases unattainable, challenge. As discussed in chapter one, until the 1990s, dentists did not really understand how to classify smiles so that they and their patients could talk the same language. Figuring out the types of smiles and which ones fit which patients, and coming up with methods for actually creating these smiles, was very difficult. By the 1990s, dentistry had a definition of the smile that finally took into account the underlying reality with respect to the face. But there remained a need for greater sophistication in analyzing and codifying different smiles and different aspects of smiles.

At this point in my own development, I was strongly affected by a paper written by the plastic surgeon R.T. Manktelow (along with J.L. Paletz and R. Chaban) and published in 1993 in *Plastic and Reconstructive Surgery*, the journal of the American Society of Plastic Surgeons. This paper, "The Shape of a Normal Smile: Implications for Facial Paralysis Reconstruction," dealt with how the angle of a smile can change. Think of lips in their resting state where the meeting of the lips is somewhat horizontal. As the smile begins, the corners of the mouth begin to shift. The degree to which they do so and at what angle, with the lips going upwards, is what creates the smile. This gave me a better insight, surgically,

Dentists needed greater sophistication in analyzing different smiles.

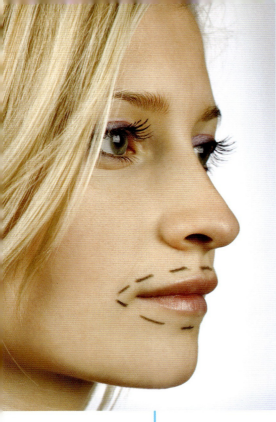

Plastic surgeons weren't looking deeply enough.

into why there is such a range in the way lips "behave" in a smile: how much they move and the angles at which they move. I saw that instead of trying to boil everything down to statistics and analysis on an individual basis, it made more sense to organize all these into patterns.

I also went back to a paper by L.R. Rubin, published in 1974, also in *Plastic and Reconstructive Surgery*. Rubin, also a plastic surgeon, was instrumental in trying to understand smile patterns. In his paper, "The Anatomy of a Smile: Its Importance in the Treatment of Facial Paralysis," he noted from surgical experience that there were various patterns to the way people smiled. He classified them as commissure, cuspid, and complex. (Hang on – we'll get to the descriptions of these patterns in a moment.)

I went on to apply the scientific findings of Manktelow to the insights of Rubin. Because both of these men were plastic surgeons, they broke the patterns they were seeing into lip movements not involving the teeth. I took their approach one step further. I said, "Okay, let's finish the story. We see how the plastic surgeon is looking at the lips. Now let's examine how the teeth follow these patterns."

I began to examine how there were patterns of angles unique to each smile. This is the essential point. By identifying the pattern, one can know the angle of smile that should be occurring but that may not be doing so because the underlying teeth are broken or have worn down. Fixing the teeth so they follow the angles of the smile pattern creates the right smile architecturally. This was the answer. If I had to pick one thing in my life that I got right, this would be it.

Because the commissure smile was the most common pattern of smile, that's the type of smile most patients were asking for and most dentists were seeking to create. But this decidedly did not work for patients whose smile patterns were not commissure.

Rubin didn't understand why the exact same surgery used to correct the smile of a car accident victim or a patient who had had a tumor removed yielded such different results. He, too, was trying to build everyone into a commissure. Plastic surgeons would lift the muscle and replace it and put it back the same way for both patients. Sometimes it worked well and the patient would feel that the surgery was very successful. But other times a patient undergoing this same surgery felt their smile was not right – in fact, that the surgery had made them look as if they weren't smiling properly. Perhaps one side of the face was smiling and the other side seemed to be leering.

After doing further research, however, Rubin was able to identify that the way a person's smile works is similar

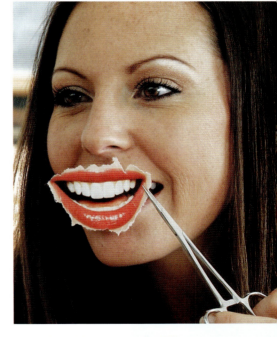

The same surgical procedure had wildly different results.

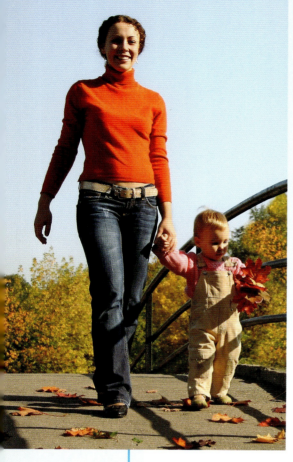

The way a smile works is similar to the way a person's walk works.

to the way a person's walk works. Two people of the same size and with similar physiques and even speeds of walking nevertheless can walk in very different ways. They may have different gaits: different speeds at "takeoff," lengths of strides, angles of knees and feet, and so on – a kind of walking signature. Some people begin their walk slowly and then pick up speed; some start off fast and maintain their speed. Some take quick short steps; others cover ground with big, strong strides. John Wayne had a characteristic way of strolling onto the movie screen. You instantly knew who it was even if you couldn't see his face. You can even tell a whole family by the similarity of their walks.

In the same way, two people with the same basic facial characteristics may have very different smiles. Some begin their smiles with their mouths closed, while others are half-way into their smile from the beginning because their mouths are already partly open. Some show little gum because their smiles are gradual and modest. Others show a lot of gum, and fast, because their smiles go quickly from liftoff to orbit.

People can alter the way they smile, but they will almost always revert to their natural smile. That's how their facial muscles do it. It is fundamentally unchangeable.

Smile Patterns

As mentioned above, there are millions of different smiles – essentially as many as there are individuals – three basic smile patterns have been identified. Plastic surgeons given the task of rehabilitating smiles have identified three neuromuscular smile patterns, the commissure, cuspid, and complex patterns.

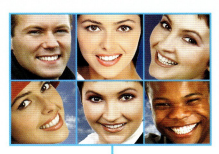

Commissure Smiles

The commissure smile is the most common pattern, seen in approximately 67% of the population. In this smile, typically thought of as a Cupid's bow, the corners of the mouth are first pulled up and outward, followed by the levators (muscles) of the upper lip contracting to show the upper teeth. The lowest incisal edge of the maxillary (upper) teeth are the central incisors. From this point, the convexity continues superiorly with the maxillary first molar being 1 to 3 mm higher than the incisal edge of the centrals. A spontaneous commissure smile results in a maximum movement of the commissure from 7 to 22 mm. Likewise, the average direction of movement of the commissure is 40 degrees from the horizontal (range 24 to 38 degrees).

For personalities with recognizable commissure smiles, think of Sienna Miller, Paris Hilton, Drew Barrymore, and Jennifer Lopez.

There are millions of different smiles.

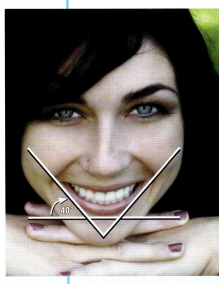

The commissure smile is the most common.

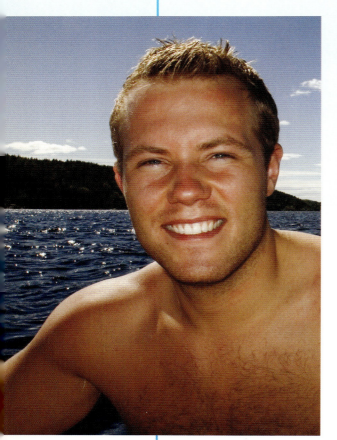

The cuspid smile is found in approximately 31% of the population.

Cuspid Smiles

The cuspid smile is found in approximately 31% of the population. In this smile, the shape of the lips is commonly visualized as a diamond. This smile pattern is identified by the dominance of the levator labii superioris. They contract first, exposing the cuspid teeth. Then the corners of the mouth contract secondarily to pull the lips upward and outward. The corners do not move as much as they do in the commissure smile. The corners of the mouth are often inferior to the height of the lip above the maxillary cuspids.

Often, in this smile pattern, there is a similar inferior turn of the maxillary premolars as opposed to the continuous convexity of a commissure smile. This "gull wing" effect is silhouetted by the gingival tissues, which correspondingly mimic the shape of the upper lip.

In cuspid smiles the maxillary molars are often at or below the incisal edge of the central incisors.

Celebrities with this pattern include Eva Longoria, Angelina Jolie, Tom Cruise, and Jennifer Aniston.

Complex Smiles

The complex smile is found in only about 2% of the population. Both upper and lower lip are actively pulled during smiling. The levators of the upper lip, the levators of the corners of the mouth, and the depressors of the lower lip contract simultaneously, showing all of the upper and lower teeth concurrently.

The key characteristic of this smile is the strong muscular pull and retraction of the lower lip downward and back. In this pattern, both maxillary and mandibular occlusal planes are generally parallel, like two chevrons.

For celebrated personalities with complex smiles, consider Julia Roberts, Oprah Winfrey, Cameron Diaz, and Britney Spears.

The Stages of a Smile

It's important to realize that a smile moves. It animates. It's not like a cavity, which is static and does not change before the dentist's eye (let's hope not, anyway). Gum disease stays the same, regardless of whether the person is talking or not talking. A smile is dynamic. You can't look at patients with their lips closed and predict what they are going to look like when they smile.

So when we're analyzing smiles, we have to look at four parts of the smile cycle: (I) The look when the

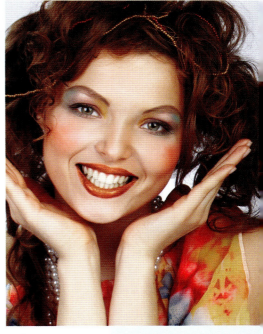

The complex smile is found in only about 2% of the population.

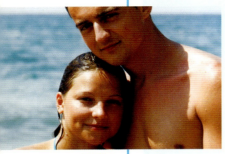
STAGE I

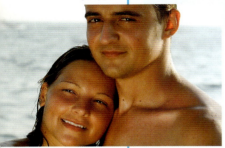
STAGE II

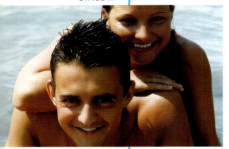
STAGE III

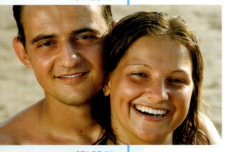
STAGE IV

Her smile is moving through four stages.

patient's lips are together. (II) The look when their lips are slightly parted – and how much tooth is showing. (III) The look when it's what we would call a normal smile – the three-quarters smile, the not quite full smile people use when being photographed. (IV) The look when the smile is exaggerated and wide, when someone is laughing wholeheartedly. These four stages are therefore termed:

Stage I	*lips closed*
Stage II	*resting display*
Stage III	*natural smile (three-quarters)*
Stage IV	*expanded smile (full)*

Dentists can use these stages to describe what the smile would look like at various points in the smile cycle. What matters is not just the smile once it has been achieved, but the whole progression of the smile, from the closed, resting stage to the fully expanded stage. I call this animation.

Of course, smiles vary and are unique to each individual. Many smiles do not differ much from a natural smile to an expanded smile. In these cases, treatment can often be restricted to the maxillary or mandibular anterior front six teeth. Other smiles differ greatly between these two stages, in which case the treatment plan to aesthetically improve the smile must be extended to a greater number of teeth.

Types of Smiles

So whenever we talk about a smile or a particular smile problem, we first have to decide, when looking at the smile, whether it is at stage I, II, III, or IV. However, when we are looking at a particular stage, we have to determine what is visible for that person within that stage. So after identifying the pattern and breaking it into stages, we have to move to the next element: identifying exactly what we are seeing at each stage.

Which brings us to smile types.

Categorizing smiles shows that there aren't an infinite number of them. There are only a certain number of variables involved. Types of smiles have to be defined based on what is showing, in terms of the upper and lower teeth, at any one time.

There are only five variations in which dental and/or periodontal tissues are displayed in what I call the smile zone – the pattern and stages together:

Type 1   *maxillary (upper jaw) only*
Type 2   *maxillary and over 3 mm gingival*
Type 3   *mandibular (lower jaw) only*
Type 4   *maxillary and mandibular*
Type 5   *neither maxillary nor mandibular*

In the vast majority of cases, people may be categorized under a single type, although there are instances in which types are combined.

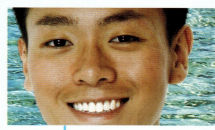
TYPE 1

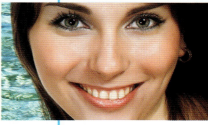
TYPE 2

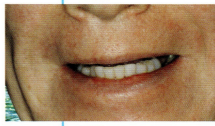
TYPE 3

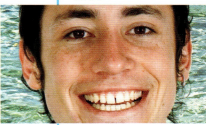
TYPE 4

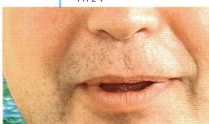
TYPE 5

There are five smile types.

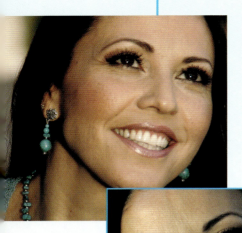

The stage of smile can change the type.

For instance, a patient may have a complex smile prominently showing maxillary and mandibular teeth and have a maxillary "gummy" smile displaying more than 3 mm of gingival tissue. This odd smile pattern would be a type 2/4.

Sometimes a change from one stage to another can change a smile's type. This woman's smile (top photo) is a type 1 in stage III, showing little gum, but (middle photo) is a type 2 in stage IV, showing a lot of gum.

Classifying Smiles

The categories above may be systematically combined to create a standardization of terms objectively describing various smiles. Pattern, stage, and type together provide a complete, easy, and concise description of smiles.

Using this system, a dentist can easily analyze and classify a particular patient's smile.

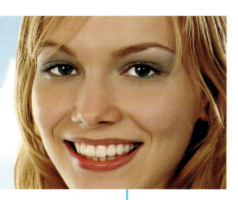

Our cover girl has a commissure smile, stage III, type 1.

Let's say you show a dentist a picture of a smile you would like. The dentist can look at it and say it's a cuspid smile, stage I, type 2. Then the dentist can analyze your actual smile to see if the desired smile fits the realities of your smile pattern.

smileline #3

THE MALE MODEL AND THE WOMAN WITH TWO SMILES

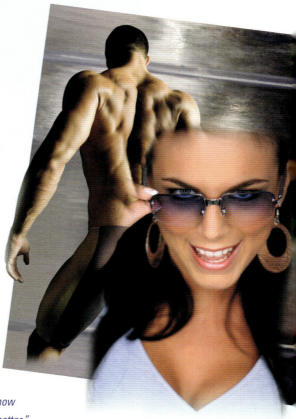

Some patients know themselves very well and have a clear idea of the smile they want. It's the dentist who's mystified.

For example, a male model came in to see me because he didn't like his smile in a basketball advertisement he was in. "I look too rugged in this photo," he said.

This short-circuited my expectations. I would have thought he wanted a more rugged look. When I mentioned my reservations to him, he became even more definite.

"No, no, I don't want to have such a rugged look," he said. "It's not appealing. People will typecast me as a rough sort of model. I need you to soften my smile."

We went through the usual consultation and I performed the procedure.

Just before he left the office, I said to him, "When you get the photos from your next shoot, show them to me and let me know if you like your smile better."

He came in a few weeks later. "I think you can handle this," he said, placing a photo on my desk with a flourish.

I couldn't believe it. The guy was short-circuiting me again. There, looking up at me from the photo, was a beautiful woman with a gorgeous smile.

"I don't understand," I said. "Why are you showing me this?"

"That's me," he said, "and that's the smile you gave me. I'm probably the country's number-one crossdresser. I do it professionally."

Another unexpected situation happened when a female patient wanted two very different smiles.

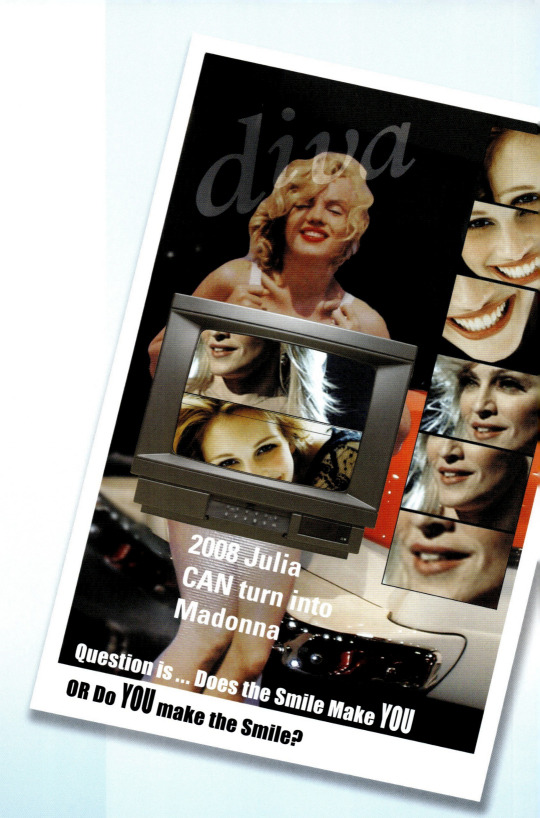

"I want a smile like Julia Roberts," was her first request. We got photos of the actress and figured out the patterns and principles of her smile to see if we could incorporate them into this patient's smile. We were pleased with the results. In fact, we even considered it a showcase example of what was possible in cosmetic dentistry.

Two years later, however, she came back and said she was dissatisfied with her smile and wanted a new one.

I confess I was a bit upset. I thought she was suggesting I had done something wrong. I was just launching into my defense when she interrupted me.

"Oh no," she said. "I love what you've done. But I no longer like Julia Roberts."

"What are you thinking of now?" I asked her with more than a little trepidation. She put a photograph down on my desk as if she was throwing down the gauntlet. The photo was of the singer Madonna.

Now, Julia Roberts and Madonna are equally outstanding in their looks – it's just that each is outstanding in her own very different way. There isn't a soul on the planet who would say the two have a striking resemblance to each other, or much resemblance at all. To make things worse, Madonna has a noticeable space between her two front teeth, whereas my patient had gone through orthodontic work and had no space between hers.

We did find, however, that a Madonna smile would work. We performed the procedure and the old Julia was very happy to be the new Madonna.

As for me, the whole experience has definitely changed my taste in entertainment. You could say I've become the number-one fan of the former Louise Ciccone of Michigan. I can't get enough of her singing and dancing. I admire her fashion sense. I'm even going to go out on a limb here and say she's one of the great actresses of our time. It's all just my way of making sure that she never falls out of favor with the public – or with her biggest fan on my patient list.

smileline #3

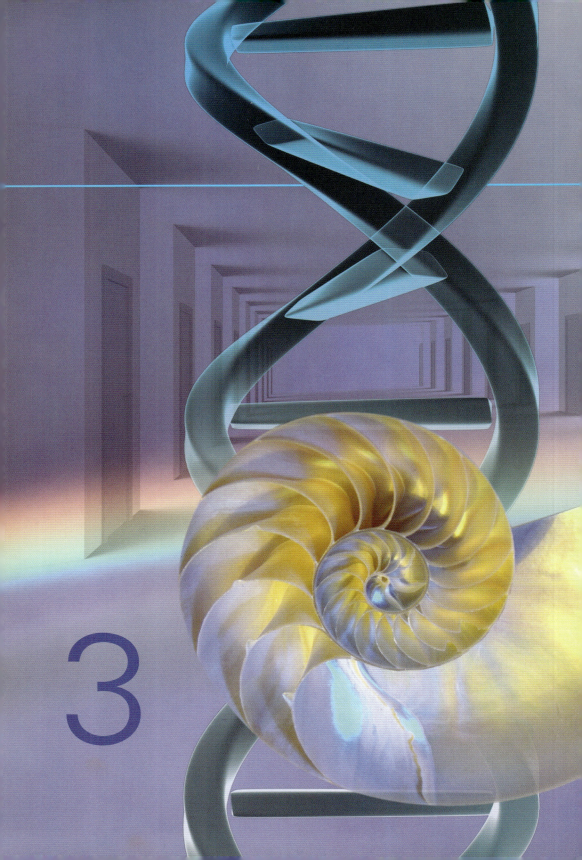

The *Big* Picture

Dentistry and the Aesthetic Principles of Nature

OUR APPRECIATION OF HUMAN BEAUTY, in contrast to our appreciation of art, has not changed significantly since ancient times. Good thing, too, because otherwise the paparazzi would be jostling each other for shots of people who looked as if they had walked out of a painting in the Museum of Modern Art. Happily, they chase after Julia Roberts, Angelina Jolie, and Charlize Theron, instead – goddesses who light up our screens and our lives with their dazzling smiles.

Aesthetics and the Laws of Nature

I cannot believe how often dentists – and I have been guilty of this, too – miss the big picture. We are tempted to focus on the teeth and the mechanics of how to fix them, failing to see that the teeth have a direct bearing on the beauty of people's smiles through their relationship to the dynamics of the face.

I find this lack of a broader vision frustrating. People who study architecture are excited by the adventurous designs of new buildings. Experienced gardeners glow when they walk past a well-landscaped lawn.

Virtually all of us, whatever our background or education, know beauty when we see it.

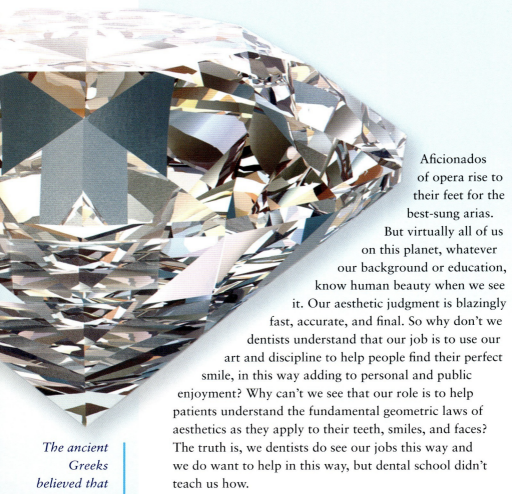

The ancient Greeks believed that art mirrors qualities that are mathematically built right into nature.

Aficionados of opera rise to their feet for the best-sung arias. But virtually all of us on this planet, whatever our background or education, know human beauty when we see it. Our aesthetic judgment is blazingly fast, accurate, and final. So why don't we dentists understand that our job is to use our art and discipline to help people find their perfect smile, in this way adding to personal and public enjoyment? Why can't we see that our role is to help patients understand the fundamental geometric laws of aesthetics as they apply to their teeth, smiles, and faces? The truth is, we dentists do see our jobs this way and we do want to help in this way, but dental school didn't teach us how.

Dentists traditionally regard aesthetics as an artistic, not a dental, concept. But we are coming to a new understanding. We must realize that there are principles behind aesthetics that can be quantified scientifically and therefore come into play in cosmetic and aesthetic dentistry. Dental aesthetics are governed by mathematical parameters. These parameters, or geometric laws, should not be viewed as immutable but as useful guidelines. When the parameters are properly applied by clinicians and laboratory technicians, restorations of unique aesthetic value may be achieved.

The job of dentists, therefore, is twofold. First, we must ensure that the teeth, as they are related to the face, are properly proportioned and conform to the laws of nature. Second, we must take the next, practical step of quantifying and qualifying what the eye sees as being pleasing smiles.

What makes a smile beautiful is not purely subjective. Ask people to vote on the quality of various smiles and you will not get wildly varying responses. In fact, it turns out that in our responses to beauty, we are real-life proof of the accuracy of the ancient Greeks' aesthetic theories. They believed that art mirrors qualities that are mathematically built right into nature. Our enjoyment of proportion and grace, therefore, appears to be innate to the way things are. Some things we find pleasing and other things not. Our reactions are not accidental but are anchored in nature itself and the artistic sense that is related to the "nature of nature."

Patients themselves may have subjective opinions about what they want, but it is the dentist's job to show them, based on aesthetic and physical principles, that there is something objective to be sought. The perfect smile is the perfect smile *for them*, given not only what they want, or even think they want, but also what they *should* want.

Let's look further at "the aesthetics of nature" and how these principles relate to the smile.

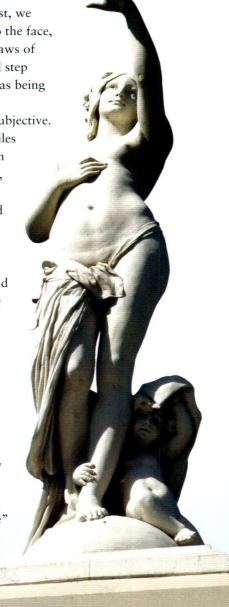

Phi: The Golden Mean

Science continues to follow the Greeks' lead.

The ancient Greeks, in investigating nature and extrapolating their findings to the study of art and architecture, developed the concept of the Golden Mean. The Greeks used this concept to name the pleasing proportion they found throughout nature of 1 to 1.6, expressed mathematically in the irrational number, 1.618033989. This concept is known by many names, including the Golden Section, the Golden Proportion, the Golden Ratio, the Perfect Division, Phi, or simply the Greek letter ø. I will use the terms "Phi" and "Golden Mean."

More than two thousand years later, science continues to follow the Greeks' lead. Nature's use of the Golden Mean can be found in the animal, vegetable, and mineral kingdoms. Nothing appears to be so small or insignificant that it does not merit a pleasing proportion. Note, for example, the endlessly embellished

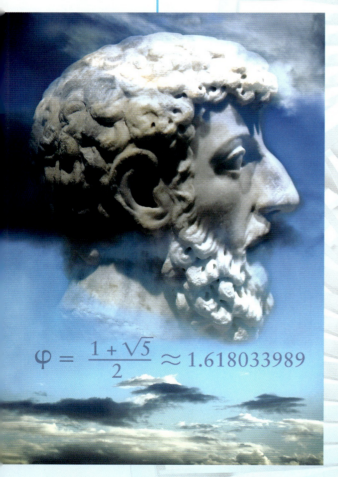

$$\varphi = \frac{1 + \sqrt{5}}{2} \approx 1.618033989$$

hexagons of the snowflake or the perfect cubes found in mineral crystals. Human beings, a remarkably symmetrical creation themselves, appear to react instinctively and positively to forms that follow rigid geometric rules, whether in nature or art.

Today we can see that even the DNA molecule, life's single most important biological structure, is in the Phi proportion. One complete revolution of the DNA double helix measures 34 angstrom. The width of the DNA helix is 21 angstrom. The ratio 34 to 21 is 1 to 1.6.

Golden Spirals

The natural form that most fully expresses the Golden Mean is nature's crowning achievement: the human body. The body begins its existence in the spiral pattern of an embryo. And when it matures, it exhibits Phi proportions in the primary relationships of its parts. The belly button divides the body, the brow divides the head, and the wrist divides the hand and forearm – all almost perfectly in the Phi proportion. Moreover, finger bones are in Phi proportion to each other, making a Golden Spiral when a fist is made. Not everyone's body exhibits perfect Phi proportions, but Phi will usually be seen as governing many of the body's key relationships.

Other examples of Golden Spirals may be found in the profile of a wave, the vortex of a tidal whirlpool, and our own solar system where the distance between the planets reflects Phi. Even the spiral of the beautiful natural nautilus shell (which is the logo of my Studio) follows the Golden Spiral.

Golden Rectangles

The 1 to 1.6 ratio has intrigued experts for centuries because of its manifestation in aesthetics. It occurs in triangles, circles, and spirals, but most notably in the Golden Rectangle, a figure with two sides bearing the magical relationship to each other. The Golden Rectangle is considered one of the most visually appealing geometric forms. For years, experts have been finding examples in everything from the edifices of ancient Greece to the best-known art masterpieces through the centuries. Even the proportions of the famous Parthenon in Greece bore

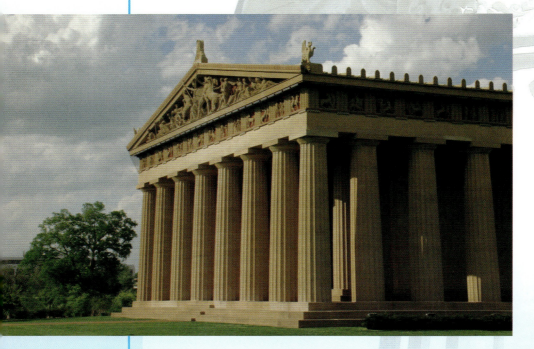

The famous Parthenon in Greece (seen here is a replica, in Nashville).

witness to the Golden Rectangle's influence.

In the thirteenth century, Thomas Aquinas, who was instrumental in resurrecting the thought of the ancient Greek philosopher, Aristotle, stated a fundamental truth about aesthetics – that "the senses delight in things duly proportioned." St. Thomas was expressing the direct and very often measurable relationship between beauty and mathematics – a relationship that applies to natural beauty and man's art.

With the knowledge that the 1 to 1.6 relationship works throughout nature, it was only a matter of time before early physicians and dentists began to opine on this relationship vis-à-vis the teeth. As dentists applied these theories to the teeth, however, a certain controversy arose. The question was whether the golden relationship was to be found in the natural, beautiful smile, as in other aspects of nature. And if it was, whether it was based on the relationship of one tooth to the other or on a general relationship of the smile relative to the overall proportions of the face.

Several of my articles argue that the answer is both – that the relationship is actually a marriage of these concepts. Dentists weren't seeing this, and for two reasons.

First, they were measuring only the relative width of teeth instead of their width in relationship to their height.

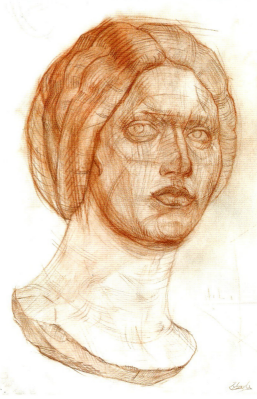

A drawing of a Greek bust, by Rune Ryberg. St. Thomas stated a fundamental truth about aesthetics, that "the senses delight in things duly proportioned."

the perfect smile

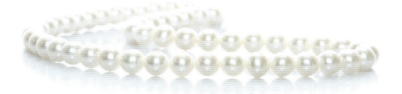

*your teeth are like
a string of pearls...*

But how can you say that something is golden by definition, mathematically, width and height, if you're only looking at the width? If the desired proportion is 1 to 1.6 and you're dealing with a very long tooth in one person's mouth, surely it can't have the same width proportion as a very short tooth in someone else's mouth.

Second, they were measuring the teeth individually instead of in relation to each other. My work showed that the two front top teeth, when viewed together as a unit, are golden in proportion, with a width-to-height ratio of 1 to 1.6. Once you've got these two teeth figured out as a Golden Rectangle, you can show their relationship to the other teeth and the overall relationship that the teeth will have to the smile and the face.

The top two front teeth are golden as a unit.

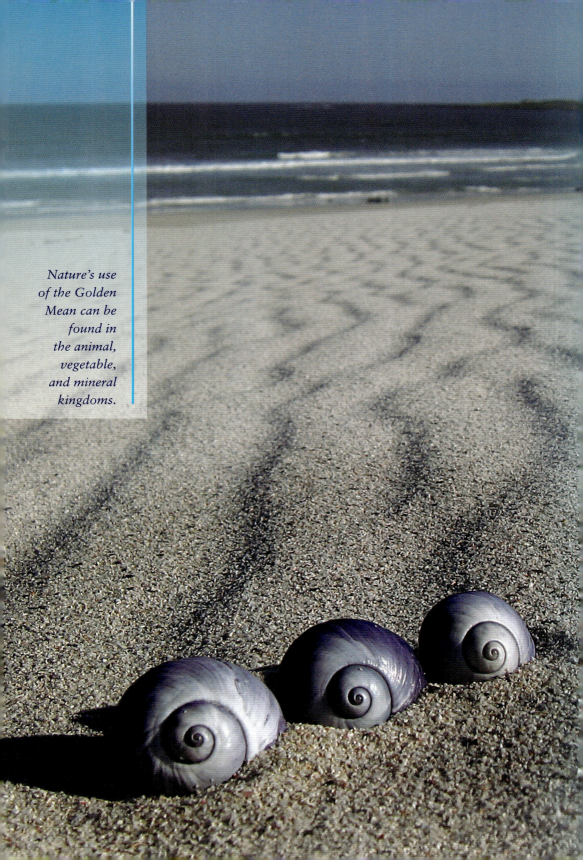

Nature's use of the Golden Mean can be found in the animal, vegetable, and mineral kingdoms.

A CLEARLY PERFECT SMILE

*It won't be long till happiness steps out to greet me.
Raindrops keep fallin' on ... my lips.*

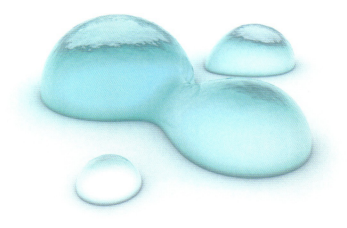

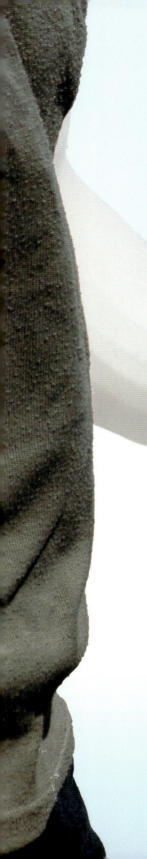

smileline #4

WHEN BEAUTY IS IN THE MIND OF THE BEHOLDER

People like to say that beauty is in the eye of the beholder – that it's just a matter of personal taste. I disagree. I think the ancient Greeks had it right when they said that beauty is built right into the way nature works.

I have been in situations, however, where beauty was definitely in the mind of the beholder. Some patients are blissfully unconcerned about the scientific and aesthetic principles of beauty. They have their own sometimes very odd notions of the kind of smile that will look good on them.

Quite a while ago now, Nancy came in for a consultation. I explained the principles of smile design in great detail and told her what I thought her smile should be.

"I really appreciate your vision," she said, "but at the end of the day, it's not what I want. In fact, I can tell you exactly what I want."

Whereupon Nancy pulled out a file with several sheets of graphics paper – the kind architects used before the days of computer-assisted design – with pictures of beautiful smiles clipped to them.

My own smile froze when she said she had narrowed her search down to a smile like Heather Locklear's.

Wrong, wrong, wrong! I had to keep from clutching my head in disbelief. Why, when her own face was tapered and her mouth and teeth were small, would she pick this particular actress to emulate, this beauty whose big-toothed, big-lipped smile travels resplendently from ear to ear across two gorgeously prominent cheekbones?

I adopted a diplomatic air that Condoleezza Rice would have envied. I reinforced that I had heard her, that I understood what she wanted. Then I segued into the gentle but firm point that what she wanted was not architecturally correct for her.

No reaction. I shifted to a more personable approach, and said, in my most caring tone, "But in this case,

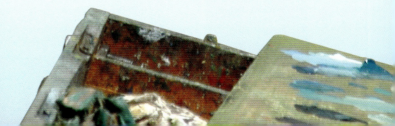

"Nancy, I'm really worried …"

"It's not Nancy, it's Nansay," she said.

I realized in that instant that a woman so particular about an idiosyncratic pronunciation of a common name was not someone who could be told what she should want.

"If a Heather Locklear smile is what you're really looking for, I can do that for you," I told her, "but on two conditions. One is that you will keep me as your dentist the rest of your life and never show another dentist the work I did for you. The other is that if anyone ever asks you who worked on you, you are to say you can't remember."

Nancy – I mean Nansay – agreed, and she's been true to her word in the decade-plus since. What's more, she is thrilled with her smile to this very day.

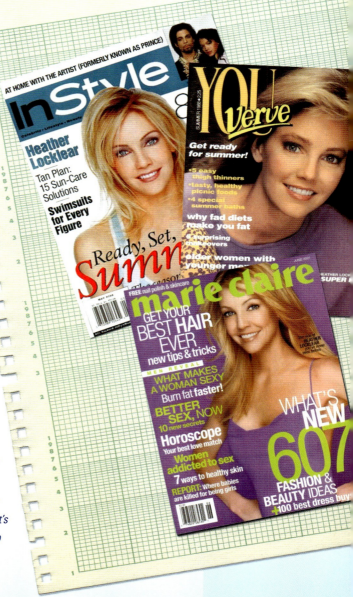

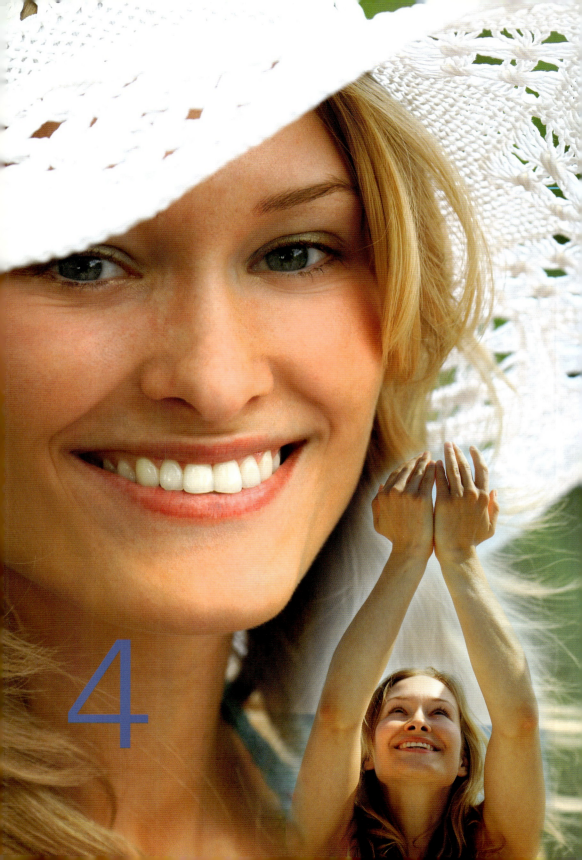

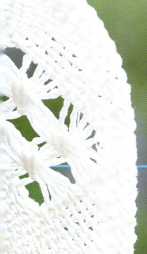

Your Once and Future Smile

Score Your Smile on the Ten Principles of Smile Design

In the previous chapter we looked at some of the fundamental principles of design. We saw how the eye responds positively to forms in nature that exhibit the "golden" proportions of geometry. And from there we looked at how those geometrical relationships form the foundation of beautiful smiles.

Now it's time to determine in more detail how the theory of design applies to actual smiles, and to develop principles of design that can be applied in practical ways by dentists. With that in mind, let's look at the ten major principles of smile design. After that, we will conclude the chapter with a test that you and your dentist can use to score your smile. The results may lead you to begin your own search for your perfect smile.

#1 The Smile Line

The smile line is described by most dentists as involving the upper six front teeth against the lower lip. (I usually call these teeth the "social six.") Although this relationship is generally true, I have observed that the progression of

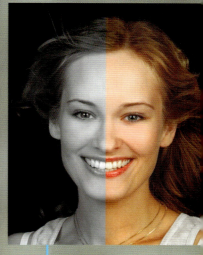

We have to look first at the patient's smile pattern.

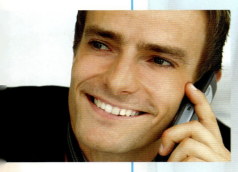

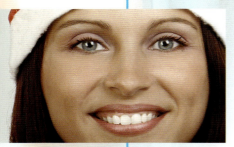

Although both smiles are not ideal, at least his smile line follows his smile pattern; hers does not follow her pattern.

the other teeth and the angles at which they follow, contrasted by the lips, must also be described, and these will not be the same for everyone. The rest of a person's smile will animate differently based on whether their smile pattern is commissure, cuspid, or complex. See chapter two for descriptions of these different smile patterns.

Not everyone has a convex smile line. In fact, people with beautiful smiles have smile lines that follow their particular smile pattern. So the first principle is that your smile line needs to mirror, or as I like to put it, silhouette, your smile pattern.

Once you or your dentist have identified your smile pattern, you can check in a mirror to see whether your smile line follows that pattern. There is no universal smile. Dentists are often told by patients, "I've had my teeth done and they look horrible on me. What happened?" The answer, in many cases, is that they may have been given a smile that does not silhouette their pattern. It's similar to fashion – for example, checkered, double-breasted jackets may not be the best choice for short men.

#2 Relative Dental Proportions

In a beautiful smile, the teeth are proportionate in two ways. First, in and of themselves, with each tooth having its own unique proportionate shape and form. And second, in how they fit with their adjacent teeth to be viewed collectively as one smile. What this means, for example, is that the maxillary front incisor should, first, be 20% taller

THE PERFECT SMILE NEVER CHANGES...

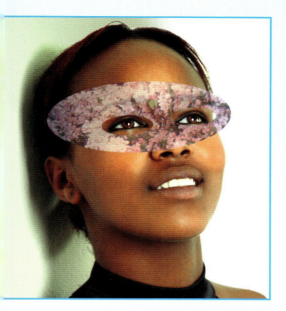
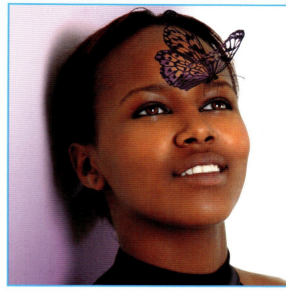

spring – cool   *summer – hot*

fall – warm   *winter – cold*

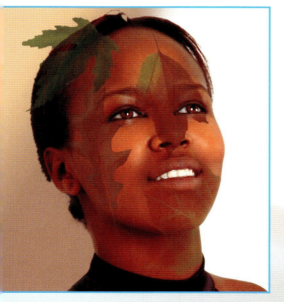
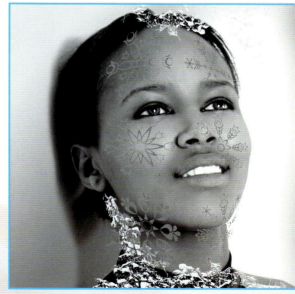

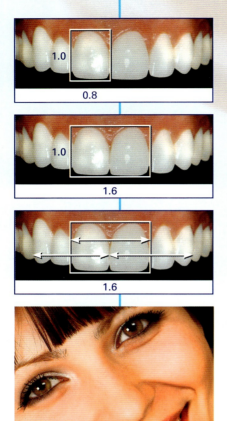

#2 Relative Dental Proportions

than it is wide. Second, the two maxillary front incisors need to be viewed as one collective unit and have a width-to-height ratio of 1 to 1.6. If the average person has a tooth that is 10 mm in height, the width of the two teeth together should be 16 mm.

Generally, as you look at your teeth straight on, your widest and longest teeth should be the two top front teeth at the midline. To the eye, the rest of the teeth should diminish in size as they cascade toward the back. I say "to the eye," because if you actually removed the cheeks and looked at the teeth straight on, a molar may in fact be wider than a front tooth – it just looks smaller at the angle from which it is usually seen. Sometimes you see a person whose back teeth look too big. Their smile does not look right because those teeth do not cascade to appear smaller as the eye looks down the smile line.

#3 Dominance of Maxillary Central Incisors

The first thing the eye focuses on when it looks at a smile are the two upper front teeth – the maxillary central incisors – together as one. If the eye does not accept these two teeth properly, it assumes that something is wrong with the whole smile. These two teeth have to work as a unit. The eye of the viewer of the smile will be thrown off if they don't match – if one is twisted or shorter, for example. People looking at such a smile automatically begin to scan left and right, picking up all of the other differences. (Interestingly, two well-proportioned front teeth will to a large extent make up for crookedness in the other teeth.)

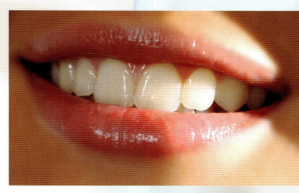

#3 Dominance of Maxillary Central Incisors

Going back briefly to our discussion of the Golden Mean in the previous chapter, it becomes clear why the central incisors are a norm that is critical to our perception of a smile. A central incisor that has an 80% width-to-height ratio is in a 1 to .8 relationship. However, the two central incisors together form a Golden Rectangle, with the coveted Phi factor of 1 to 1.6.

A pleasing smile, therefore, must have maxillary incisors that dominate the smile. This principle advocates an ideal width-to-height for the maxillary central incisor. Interestingly, these are the only two teeth in the entire smile for which mirror-image symmetry is a must.

Note that the height of teeth can change over time. An unworn tooth may actually be 75% width to height. But because some wear is common, we use 80% as the standard, which is actually a shorter tooth, width to height. Height can appear to change because of changes to the gum line, as well, thus creating a different illusion as to the true height of the tooth.

The width of teeth, however, rarely changes. You can't floss the width of your tooth off. From the width of one central incisor, you can easily establish the desired height

FLIP YOUR SMILE

... you'll find that life is worthwhile

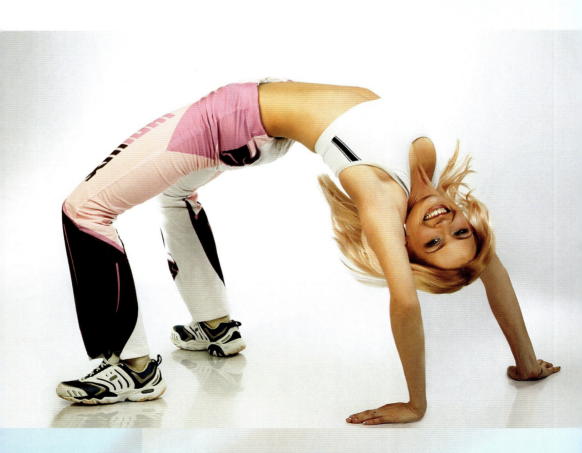

of the two teeth from gum line to incisal edge. Since these two teeth are identical, you can establish the relative dental proportions of the remaining front teeth. As mentioned, the upper teeth are critically important to the character of the smile, which is why they are called the social six.

#4 Silhouettes

There are two sets of silhouettes, an anterior one and a posterior one.

The anterior silhouette may be described as the relationship of the front upper four teeth to each other. Specifically, the particular angle or curve of the back side of your front central incisor should perfectly mirror the back angle or curve of your lateral incisor, the second tooth. If the front two teeth, the central incisors, are a mirror image of each other, this silhouette pattern will mirror on its other sides as well, creating a harmony between the front four maxillary teeth.

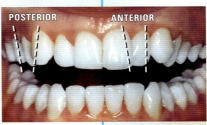
BEFORE

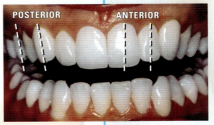
AFTER

#4 Silhouettes

The posterior silhouette may be described as the particular line angle of your cuspid, the third tooth from the midline. The angle of each tooth that follows, as you go to the teeth in the back of the mouth, the premolars and the molars, needs to mirror this line angle.

The line angles of some people's teeth range from straight to a continuous curve, or even begin straight and then end curved. But whatever shape one tooth has, the teeth that follow need to have that same silhouette.

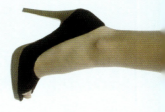

Therefore, it's not the particular line angle that's considered aesthetic but rather how the angles all silhouette together. Ideally, the anterior set of silhouettes match each other and the posterior sets of silhouettes match each other.

Patients often notice that when individual teeth are bonded, veneered, or crowned, they tend to look artificial, even when the color matches perfectly. Invariably, what the eye is seeing is a lack of this principle of silhouettes. Because these procedures are inherently adding thickness to the existing size of the tooth, the result often does not silhouette.

#5 Progression of Maxillary Incisal Embrasures

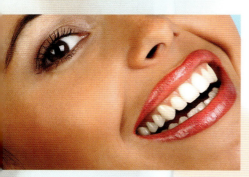

#5 Progression of Maxillary Incisal Embrasures

Incisal embrasures are the little spaces between the edges of your teeth that you can fit your nail into. There is a pattern of these embrasures that appeals to the eye. Ideally, the embrasure between the front two teeth is very small; the embrasure between the next two, the central and its lateral, is subsequently larger, about twice as big; and when you get to the third one, the embrasure between the lateral and the cuspid, it's twice as big again. So in a pleasing smile, there's a natural progression between the spaces of the teeth.

The pattern of embrasures is in fact an area where there is tremendous subjective opinion. In fact, various smile styles have various patterns for these embrasures. Often patients may like an even pattern of embrasures through-

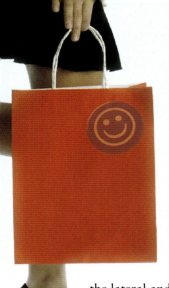

I'm shopping for a smile today!

out the teeth, or no embrasures between the front four and perhaps a pronounced embrasure between the lateral and the cuspid, to create a "sporty" look. In fact, there are no fewer than 20 common incisal embrasure patterns, and this may be the single most important subjective principle that can greatly change the design of your smile.

#6 Progression of Contacts

Not only do the incisal edges of the teeth ideally have a certain convexity, but they must also "make contact" with each other in a pleasing way. By "contact" we mean the spot that floss binds between your teeth. The point at which the teeth make contact over the social six should mirror the convexity of the smile line. In other words, a very curvaceous smile line should have contacts that curve in the same manner. A relatively flat smile line would have contacts that line up relatively evenly.

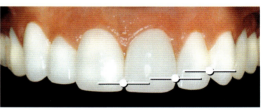

#6 Progression of Contacts

Sometimes, if a tooth has moved or shifted over time or has been filled incorrectly, it will touch the tooth next to it at the wrong spot. The difference may be subtle, but it throws off the pattern of the teeth. As already discussed in this chapter, the eye is offended when it picks up conflicting patterns.

Ideally, each contact point steps up and follows the curve of the incisal edges. As incisal edges curve, the contacts curve the same way. Sometimes a dentist will

Your Once and Future Smile

achieve the correct edge on a patient's tooth, but will get the contact on the wrong spot on the tooth. This makes the tooth look bulky or appear to be improperly placed.

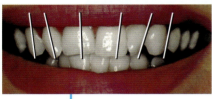

BEFORE

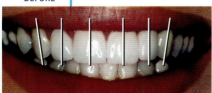

AFTER

#7 Axial Alignment

#7 Axial Alignment

The axial alignment of teeth is the pattern by which the teeth line up with each other. The teeth may sit inside the jaw in relatively different positions. They may all line up and appear to be quite vertical. They may line up and be vertical at the front, with the remaining teeth all at an angle of 5 degrees. Or they could even be like a fan where they start straight and each tooth subsequently "folds" out.

The key for the dentist is to find the pattern unique to each person. If it is determined to be a good pattern, then the dentist must make sure not to change it when they put veneers or crowns on the teeth. If it is determined to be a defective pattern, then the right one has to be determined and implemented. For example, if someone has a very angular face, you will want those teeth to have some sort of angle as the teeth cascade down.

#8 Gingival Zenith

When dentists put veneers or crowns on teeth, they of course have to follow the shape of the teeth they are treating. But they also have to adjust the gum line to fit the teeth properly. When that isn't done, people perceive something to be wrong with the teeth, when it's the gum line, not the teeth, that's the problem.

The gum line around the two front teeth should have beautifully shaped curves or arches (think of the golden arches of McDonald's). After all, if the gum line was pointy or oblong, it wouldn't fit properly over those teeth. Gum lines have a unique shape for each tooth. The maxillary central incisor has a different shape from that of the lateral incisor and from that of the cuspid. The shape of the curve above the teeth has certain high points. Each particular point is called a gingival zenith.

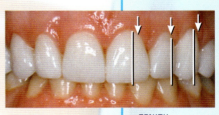

ZENITH

GAL

#8 Gingival Zenith

The placement of the zenith can be highly critical to making the overall portion of the tooth look natural to the gum. Today, changes to the gum line are easily adjusted with dental lasers.

#9 Occlusion

If your occlusion – your bite – isn't right, it's going to change the dynamics of how your smile, and you, look.

Bite is important. Orthodontists have clearly shown that because your face is wider at your mid-part than at your chin, your upper jaw should be larger than your lower jaw and all the upper teeth should umbrella your lower teeth. This is often not the case. Consider some of the potential disharmonies that we may inherit:

- The genes we get for our lower jaw may be different from the set of genes we get for our upper jaw.

Your Once and Future Smile

- The genes we get for our teeth may be different from those we get for our jaws.

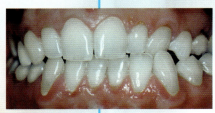

BEFORE

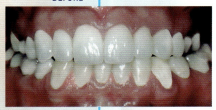

AFTER

#9 *Occlusion*

- The jaws may not match each other. The teeth inside will therefore not be the right match for the jaws.
- When the lower jaw sticks out farther than the upper jaw, it sets the teeth on the opposite side, which we call a cross bite, and this looks prognathic (prominent). In the animal kingdom – alligators or dogs, for instance – the lower jaw is obviously bigger than the upper jaw. Fortunately, this is rare in humans.
- When the upper jaw sticks out farther than the lower jaw, the result is what we call buck teeth, which we consider architecturally unacceptable.

#10 *Color*

The ideal color of your teeth must be considered in relation to your skin tone. There is a view in dentistry that your teeth should be as white as the whites of your eyes, but this is a myth. There is no such thing as the right color. It is actually a subjective consideration. If you applied the zinc ointment that clowns use to your face, your teeth would instantly look brown. As soon as you washed the ointment off, they would look whiter.

Studies have been done in which thousands of teeth were analyzed by different dental practitioners who were

#10 Color

compiling professional work on the anatomy of teeth. It is often thought that darker people have whiter teeth, but once the teeth were on the table, their racial origin could not be discerned.

Basically, your teeth need to be relatively lighter than your skin tone. Either get them whitened or wear more makeup or get a sun tan. We will examine various methods for lightening teeth in the following chapter.

At times, more than one principle can apply to an area of teeth. Ensure that in fact the correction of one principle does not trigger the misalignment of another.

A Revolutionary Test

So enough with design theory. Now let's put it into practice. What follows is revolutionary – a test with which you can actually score your own smile against the ten smile principles discussed above. Doing this will arm you with the "evidence" you need in pursuing your perfect smile through dental treatment.

You can score your smile on your own or with a friend – or better yet, with your dentist. Just follow the directions to find out your score.

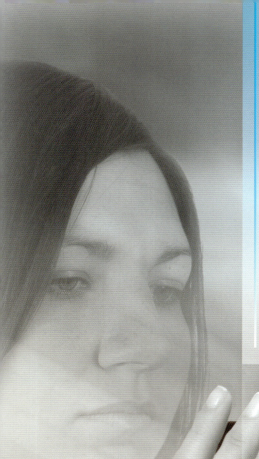

Scoring Your Smile
Using the mDAI

Score your smile by rating it on each of the ten smile principles discussed in this chapter, using the Modified Dental Aesthetic Index. Here's how you do it: If your smile is excellent on an individual principle of smile design, give it a score of 10. If it is acceptable but not excellent, give it a score of 5. If it's not acceptable at all, give it a score of 0. Then add up your scores.

- If everything about your smile is perfect (and if it is, you are probably working in Hollywood and shouldn't be reading this book), your score will add up to 100.
- If you've got a really good smile, you're going to have a score of over 70, which means there is still room for improvement.
- If your smile gets a score lower than 50, you definitely need to consider having work done on your smile.

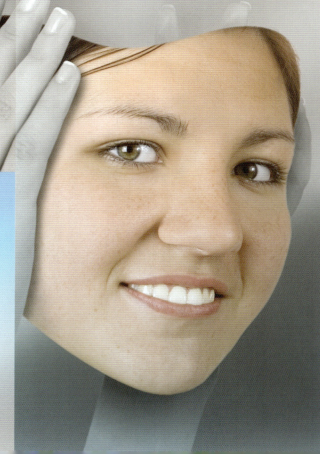

Modified Dental Aesthetic Index Scale

1. The Smile Line
2. Relative Dental Proportions
3. Dominance of Maxillary Central Incisors
4. Silhouettes
5. Progression of Maxillary Incisal Embrasures
6. Progression of Contacts
7. Axial Alignment
8. Gingival Zenith
9. Occlusion
10. Color

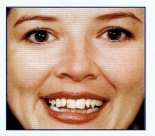
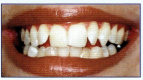
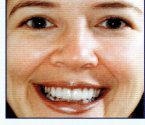
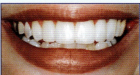

Before		After
0	The Smile Line	10
0	Dental Proportions	10
5	Dominance	10
0	Silhouettes	5
0	Embrasures	10
0	Contacts	10
5	Axial Alignment	5
10	Gingival Zenith	10
10	Occlusion	10
10	Color	10
40	**mDAI total**	**90**

Score changed from mDAI = 40 to mDAI = 90

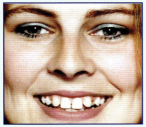
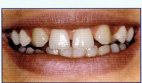
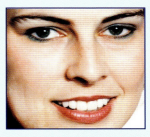
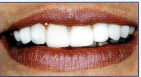

Before		After
0	The Smile Line	10
0	Dental Proportions	10
5	Dominance	10
0	Silhouettes	10
0	Embrasures	10
0	Contacts	10
5	Axial Alignment	5
5	Gingival Zenith	5
10	Occlusion	10
10	Color	10
35	**mDAI total**	**90**

Score changed from mDAI = 35 to mDAI = 90

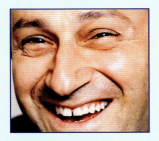
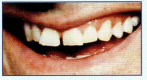
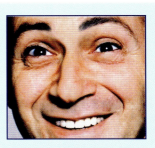
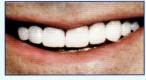

Before		After
0	The Smile Line	10
0	Dental Proportions	10
5	Dominance	10
5	Silhouettes	5
0	Embrasures	10
5	Contacts	10
0	Axial Alignment	5
5	Gingival Zenith	10
10	Occlusion	10
5	Color	10
35	**mDAI total**	**90**

Score changed from mDAI = 35 to mDAI = 90

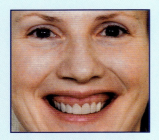
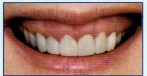

Before		After
0	The Smile Line	10
5	Dental Proportions	10
10	Dominance	10
5	Silhouettes	10
10	Embrasures	10
10	Contacts	10
5	Axial Alignment	5
0	Gingival Zenith	5
10	Occlusion	10
5	Color	10
60	mDAI total	90

Score changed from mDAI = 60 to mDAI = 90

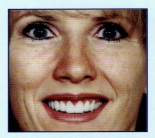
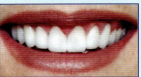

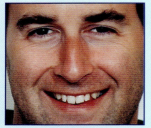
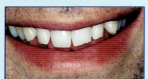

Before		After
5	The Smile Line	10
5	Dental Proportions	10
0	Dominance	10
5	Silhouettes	10
0	Embrasures	10
5	Contacts	10
5	Axial Alignment	10
10	Gingival Zenith	10
10	Occlusion	10
10	Color	5
55	mDAI total	95

Score changed from mDAI = 55 to mDAI = 95

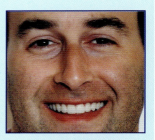
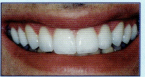

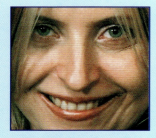
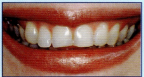

Before		After
5	The Smile Line	10
5	Dental Proportions	10
5	Dominance	10
5	Silhouettes	10
5	Embrasures	10
5	Contacts	10
5	Axial Alignment	10
5	Gingival Zenith	5
10	Occlusion	10
5	Color	10
55	mDAI total	95

Score changed from mDAI = 55 to mDAI = 95

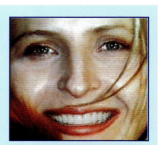
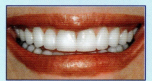

smileline #5

SIGNING ON
AND SIGNING OFF

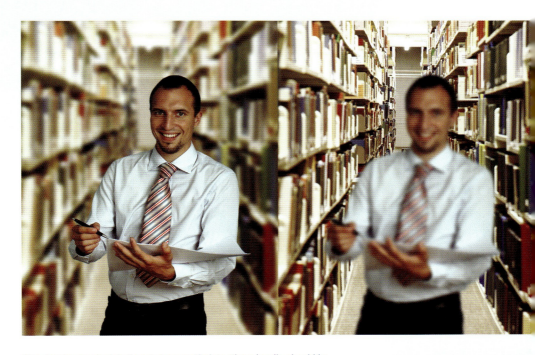

People who need a lot of work done on their teeth and smile should be very careful when making decisions with their dentists. Why? Because the tendency is for such patients to think that anything they have done is going to be an improvement. Once they see themselves looking better, however, they may very well begin to regret that they didn't have a different procedure or a more extensive one. Compare this with people who already have good teeth and smiles. They make decisions about altering their smiles more carefully because they don't want to compromise a good thing.

A tall, slim gentleman – let's call him Frank – came in for a consultation. He was six feet seven but no more than 160 pounds. At first I was very confused by Frank. No matter how he spoke or smiled, I could not see his teeth. I was beginning to think he didn't have any. But when I examined him in the chair later, I saw that he had been born with microdontia, tiny teeth genetically disproportionate to his size.

We always teach patients the ten principles of smile design, which helps us work together to choose the procedures most appropriate for them. Frank, however, seemed to pay little attention, protesting that he didn't need the seminar.

"It's just not necessary," he said. "You know what you've got to do. I've come to you and I trust you. Whatever you do is going to be of benefit."

This made us nervous, but he was resolute in his position. But sure enough, months later, he called us and said he had some concerns. Being an out-of-town patient, he could not come to see us for several months. All we could do was say that it was a big change to go from little teeth to normal teeth. "Obviously, you're going to feel they look a little odd at first," we told him.

When Frank finally came in to see us, we barely recognized him. He had put on about 75 pounds. He was obviously eating better. He seemed happier. We thought we had performed a miracle, transforming this man from sad and self-conscious to happy, healthy, and self-confident.

To our surprise, Frank proceeded to lecture us for an hour on all the design principles we thought he had ignored in our earlier session. The man was an expert ... he could have taught the course. He brought up various pattern issues and told us his embrasures were not the way he wanted them.

However, other than a few minor things, there was little we could do. He had signed off on the procedure.

Going back to your dentist the way Frank did is like building a house and then telling the architect, "You know what? I never really wanted a two-storey house."

Too much, too late.

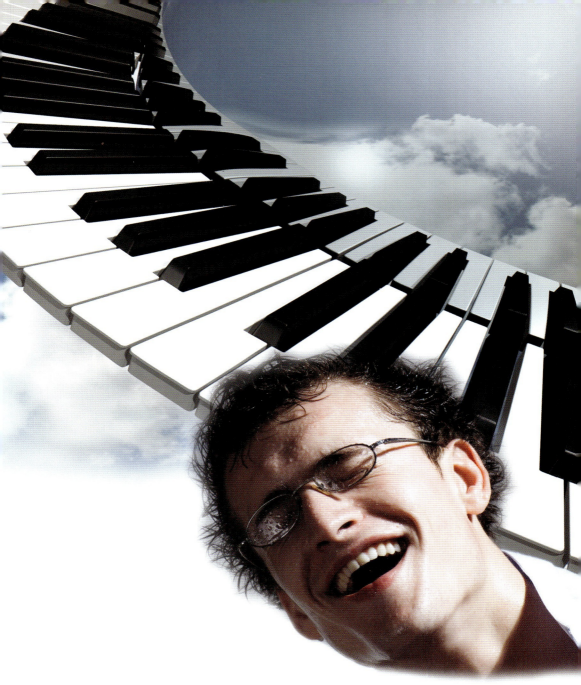

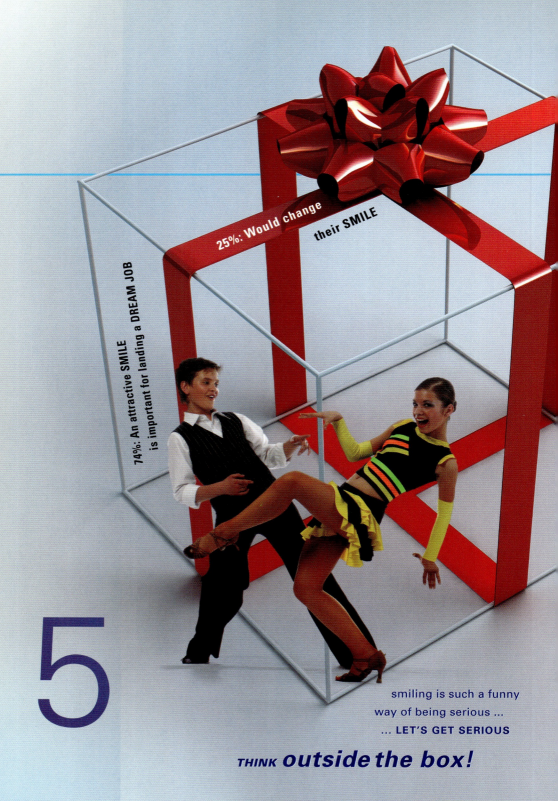

The *Fix* Is In

Solving Common Smile Problems

84%: An attractive SMILE is important for meeting MISS RIGHT

P<small>EOPLE OFTEN DISLIKE CERTAIN ASPECTS OF THEIR SMILE.</small> It's too big. It's too small. It's too *something*.

The dentist, though, needs to be able to analyze and quantify what's behind these reactions. Using the classifications and principles we've seen in previous chapters, dentists today should be able to look at smiles that are not pleasing and figure out aesthetically, mathematically, and scientifically what is wrong with them – and say to their patients, "Now *this* is what would work."

Let's look at some of the tools that can be used to fix smiles. After that, we'll examine specific smile problems and their solutions.

The Cosmetic Dentistry Toolbox

Following is quick survey of some of the products, services, and procedures currently available to dentists.

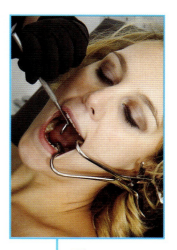

There are many tools available to dentists today.

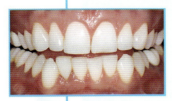

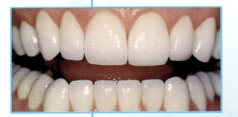

The difference veneering can make.

Veneers and Crowns

Veneers are commonly used to correct aesthetic dental problems such as defects, problems with shape, crookedness, and gaps. An advantage of applying veneers, compared with applying crowns, is that the tooth does not usually need to be ground down much to create room for the veneer. By keeping as much of the tooth structure as possible, the veneer can be quite thin over the intact, good part of the tooth, and then be thicker where the correction is needed.

Veneers are not cemented but are permanently bonded to the remaining tooth structure. As such, the refractive light properties of a veneer are similar to those of the natural tooth, creating a highly natural result. Veneers can be painted and stained to match the natural teeth, but layering is still preferred. (More on layering, later.)

Because veneers are highly transparent and bond seamlessly to the tooth, the edges of the veneers do not have to be placed underneath the gum line, which enables the health of the gum line and the natural tooth to be kept intact. This is a large advantage over crowns, which generally do go below the gum line. Crowns are inherently reflective, in order not to show the metal underneath. They are therefore extra difficult to match up properly against natural teeth. As well, should the gum line recede over time, the margin of a crown may become exposed and look unsightly.

Crowns are the treatment of choice, however, when the entire surface of the tooth is a problem but the root system is intact. Traditionally, when they were first introduced, crowns were cast and made from solid yellow gold. Today, even though they are not considered aesthetic, gold crowns continue to be the longest-term, most predictable solution.

To meet aesthetic needs, most crowns are now made from gold that is covered with tooth-colored porcelain. These porcelain-fused-to-metal crowns are the standard in most practices. However, their degree of aesthetic naturalness and beauty is highly dependent on the artistic skill of the ceramist. But there is a possibility of porcelain chipping with this type of crown, exposing the unsightly metal.

Most recently, to address the need for higher aesthetics, zirconia – which is a good replacement for metal and yet is tooth colored – has been used to eliminate the metal under the crowns and the black line or hue often seen around the edges of porcelain-fused-to-metal crowns.

Bridges

Bridges are single or multiple false teeth that are fused between two crowns on the two adjacent teeth in order to replace missing teeth. These crowns are bonded or cemented to the teeth on either side of the space.

Although bridges, to appear natural, are traditionally coated in tooth-colored porcelain on the outside, a metal underlying support is usually employed to provide strength for the bridge. Currently, zirconia is

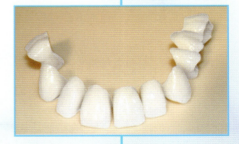

A new bridge, using teeth made of zirconia, and an old bridge, using porcelain fused to metal.

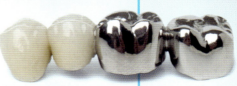

The Fix Is In   79

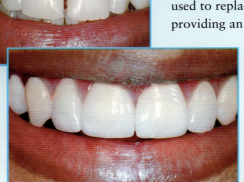

Bonding is best for minor problems.

used to replace the metal for strength, thus providing an all-tooth-colored structure.

Bonding

In the bonding procedure, composite resin is applied to the surface of a tooth and fused permanently to it. This is done to address various problems, including filling cavities, closing gaps between teeth, lengthening or widening teeth, covering dark spots, or even simply whitening teeth. Bonding is best for minor problems. If the space to be filled is very large, or little remains of the original tooth, the dentist will have to use other solutions, such as veneers, crowns, and inlays.

The term "bonding" can also refer generically to any procedure in which crowns or veneers are fused, rather than cemented, to teeth.

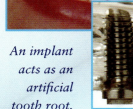

An implant acts as an artificial tooth root.

Implants

An implant is a titanium screw surgically placed into the jawbone where a tooth is missing. The implant acts as an artificial tooth root. A new tooth can then be attached to the implant.

Implants can enhance a smile by replacing missing teeth. For the implants to be attached successfully, patients must have enough bone in the area of the missing teeth.

Porcelain

Porcelain describes a family of materials used to fashion crowns and veneers. Porcelain looks very natural because it captures and reflects light like a real tooth. What we call porcelain is really a fusion of glass, plastic, and ceramic particles that provide color and a lifelike appearance.

Porcelain systems vary widely in their cost, appearance, quality, and applicability to different problems. Recent advances in porcelain technology allow dentists to use durable materials that closely mimic the particular light-transmission properties, textures, and colors of natural teeth.

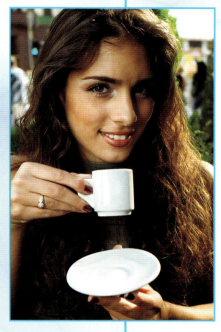

Porcelain was traditionally a hardened powder-liquid mixture, and it had limited strength. Currently, advanced porcelain systems are created from pre-pressed blocks or ingots of solid porcelain. One of the advantages of these pressed ceramics is that they can be used in cases that normally would have required the use of metal.

Porcelain looks very natural because it captures and reflects light.

Porcelains need to be colored to appear natural and match the natural teeth. They can be painted, but this can create an opacious appearance that matches the look of natural teeth only in certain light conditions. A more complicated but truer technique is to layer the porcelain with semitransparent colors, more closely mimicking the refractive properties of a natural tooth. Layering is a highly specialized ceramic art form. Its results are highly dependent on the skill of the ceramist.

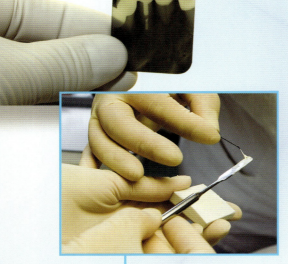

Posts can be made of metal or ceramics.

Posts

Often a tooth is so severely broken or decayed that very little of it is visible above the gum line. These teeth can nevertheless be repaired if the underlying root structure and gum are intact. Most commonly, before a crown can be fabricated, the underlying root structure is strengthened by the placement of a post, which is cemented into the former canal of the root. If the tooth is still alive, a root canal procedure may be done prior to placement of the post. Posts can be made of a metal or ceramic material, depending on aesthetic and/or strength issues.

Inlays

Inlays, also called onlays, are generally laboratory-made fillings used to repair broken or decayed premolars and molars. These fillings are made of materials that are more durable than the composite-bonding fillings traditionally used by dentists. As well, the shape of the filling is not as dependent on the dentist's skill, particularly when the filling is large. The inlay is made through a modeling process that highly improves the ability to design such restorations.

Although the inlay process traditionally requires two visits, today's CAD/CAM (computer-aided design/computer-aided manufacturing) systems enable dentists to actually machine the ceramic filling in one appointment.

CEREC

Ongoing developments in dental technology continue to make care increasingly accurate and convenient for patients. For example, patients needing a permanent all-ceramic crown, onlay, or veneer can now receive such a treatment in one visit, courtesy of a system called CEREC.

In this procedure, created by Sirona Dental Systems, the dentist first removes decayed and weakened tooth tissue, just as in other restorations. From this point on, however, things become very different. Instead of having the patient bite down into a goopy tray, the dentist coats the tooth with a non-toxic, tasteless powder. A few minutes later, a digital photograph is taken of the tooth, which the CEREC machine, prompted by special software, quickly converts into a three-dimensional virtual model. This digital information is in turn sent to a separate milling machine in the office. Ten or twenty minutes later, the restoration is ready for the dentist to fit and bond in place, followed by polishing.

Besides being used for crowns and fillings, CEREC can be employed in repairing chipped or discolored front teeth. A major advantage of this system is that it bonds ceramic materials to the tooth *chemically* rather than *mechanically*. This enables dentists to save as much healthy tooth tissue as possible.

The newest system, to be released in the market shortly, is made by a company called D4D.

Computers are more and more a part of the dentist's team.

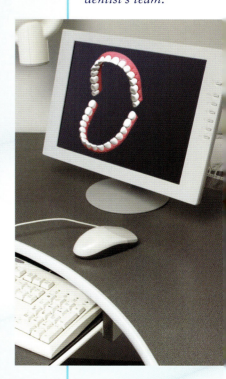

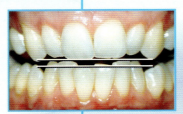

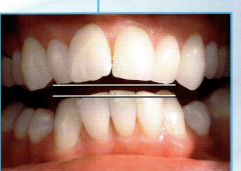

Candidates for contouring. Squint to see what the teeth would look like if countoured.

Dental Contouring

Contouring is a highly successful, though often overlooked, procedure. Many long, pointed, and chipped teeth can be easily corrected by reshaping those areas, with special diamond-impregnated drills. This sanding and polishing process, if done properly, is not harmful to the teeth.

Teeth tend to shift and drift over time, and these natural movements can actually create an improper wear pattern and possibly a cycle of continual chipping and wearing. Often a realignment of all the teeth through contouring not only improves the aesthetics greatly but also actually restores true form and function.

Whitening

The process of whitening uses bleaching substances, applied at the dentist's office or at home, to lighten the color of natural teeth. Teeth naturally darken over time, and whitening allows a patient to restore teeth to a more youthful-looking shade. Not everyone is a good candidate for whitening – for example, patients whose teeth are heavily filled.

Currently, whitening is the number-one dental procedure in North America. Its rapid popularity has left the public somewhat confused as to the various systems and claims.

There are two types of whitening: extrinsic and intrinsic.

Extrinsic whitening consists of various techniques that remove color and stains from the outside of the tooth. The whitest color that can be achieved through this method is the color achieved by a professional dental cleaning. You should assess the color of your teeth after such cleaning to see what your natural color is. If you are satisfied with this color, but over time, after the cleaning, the teeth seem to discolor, then toothpastes, mouth rinses, or another professional dental cleaning will help reestablish optimal color.

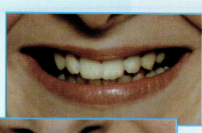

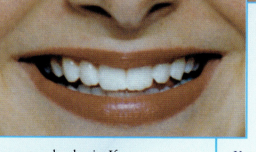

One cannot achieve, through extrinsic whitening, a result any greater than the true, inherent color of the teeth.

Intrinsic whitening is required if you find that the color of the teeth, even after a professional dental cleaning, is still too dark. In this process, the inner parts of the teeth are bleached to dissolve some of the inorganic pigments causing the discoloration.

Although there are various techniques that claim to bleach teeth intrinsically, all intrinsic whitening – whether we're talking about custom trays fabricated by dentists, over-the-counter products, strips that are applied to the teeth, or powerful lights or lasers used in a dental office –

You'll wonder where the yellow went.

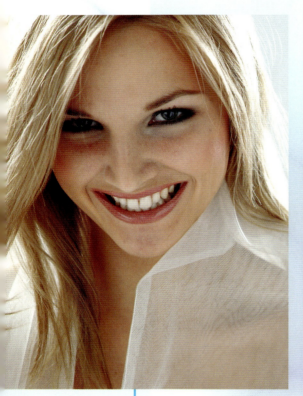

is done with the same chemical process. The only difference between the various techniques is the amount of concentration they require and the time they take.

You should customize your choice based on your personal preferences. Most people prefer the one-hour office procedure, for the sake of convenience, but studies clearly show that the results of in-office whitening are limited and have a higher rebound than the more traditional long-term process of wearing custom bleaching trays for seven to ten days.

Some patients worry about making their teeth too white by over-bleaching. The good news is that there's little danger of this. It *is* possible, however, to go too white

Your teeth should be lighter than your skin tone.

with veneers or caps. When designing a smile, the color of any artificial restorations should be carefully matched to the teeth. There is no universal right color.

As mentioned earlier, it was once thought that the color of your teeth should match the whites of your eyes. This is simply not true – tooth color is perceived relative to the color of lips, skin, and clothes. If you have pale skin, your teeth will look yellower. If you get a tan, they'll look whiter. The only real guideline is that your teeth should be lighter than your skin tone.

Root canals are the tiny nerves inside the teeth.

Root Canals

"As painful as a root canal" is a commonly used phrase. But root canal procedures, when done properly, are not painful at all.

What causes the need for this procedure? The tiny canals in teeth may become infected, which can lead to an infection in the pulp of the tooth. A dentist or endodontist performs the root canal procedure, removing the infection and later giving the tooth a filling or crown.

It is a widely held myth that a tooth that has undergone a root canal procedure has no feeling. However, the only nerve removed from the tooth in a root canal is the one that discerns heat or cold. The remaining nerves – those surrounding the tooth, where they are joined to bone and gum – continue to give the tooth feeling. So when you tap your teeth you should not be able to tell the difference between a natural tooth and a root-canalled tooth.

Gum surgery used to be relegated to correcting health issues such as gingivitis or periodontal disease.

Gum Surgery

Traditionally, gum surgery was performed to correct health issues such as gingivitis or periodontal disease – diseases that cause teeth to become infected and loosen. Correcting the gums allowed people to maintain their teeth. Today, however, gum surgery may also be used to treat aesthetic problems, without weakening the long-term viability of the teeth.

Gums will often change their shape and

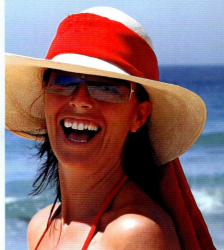

placement due to the crookedness of teeth or as a result of gumminess existing from birth.

Sometimes it's not enough, in correcting a smile, to place the teeth in the proper position – the gum line has to be corrected, too.

Dentures and Partial Dentures

Dentures are removable replacements for missing teeth. They are usually made out of a red acrylic resin, to replace gum, and white "teeth," to replace missing teeth. Chromium cobalt metal is often incorporated into the base of dentures to add structural support.

Several advantages of dentures for patients with missing teeth include strengthening the face muscles that require the support of teeth; maintaining the vertical dimension; aiding chewing; and enhancing aesthetic appearance.

If costs are a concern, consider that dentures and partial dentures can legally be made by dental therapists as well as dentists.

Samples of dentures

Orthodontics

Orthodontics is the branch of dentistry dedicated to correcting tooth alignment and bite problems. In orthodontics, the teeth and/or jaw are fitted with wires and brackets, which reposition teeth by applying pressure.

Depending on the crookedness of your teeth, you may need to see an orthodontist as part of your treatment program.

It is often thought that all of one's teeth are necessarily involved in orthodontic treatment. It's true that people undergoing this treatment usually have braces for their whole mouth, but orthodontics can be employed to move even just one tooth.

Although wires are generally used to apply the needed pressure, there is a major alternative today called Invisalign, a relatively new orthodontic technology. Instead of wire braces, Invisalign uses a series of clear, hard plastic appliances that snap into place over the teeth to gradually reposition them. A computer model predicts the step-by-step motion of the patient's teeth from their original position to their desired position. Every few weeks, a new mold is generated and sent to the patient, who simply snaps it into place.

Wires and brackets apply pressure to the teeth to reposition them.

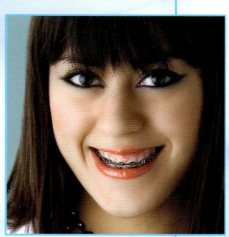

The Invisalign method offers the advantage that the appliance may be removed when desired, for eating, socializing, brushing, flossing, and so on, whereas once wires are in place, they cannot be removed until the treatment has been completed.

For major orthodontic problems, traditional wire methods are still more effective.

Like most technologies, laser technology has decreased in size and increased in strength.

Lasers in Dentistry

Laser technology is used in various aspects of dentistry. The advantage of laser therapy is the precision it offers dentists as they seek to treat very specific problems in very specific ways today. Numerous manufacturers produce various types of lasers. However, dentists and patients should be guided by the following information.

If a gingevectomy or some type of soft-tissue surgery is anticipated, the ideal wavelength of the laser is 980 nm, with the range being from 810 nm to 1064 nm.

If hard-tissue surgery is anticipated – such as surgery on teeth or bone – the ideal wavelength is in the 2780 nm to 2940 nm range.

Smile Problems and Solutions

Now that we've considered what's in the dentist's toolbox, it's time to see these materials and procedures in action. How do dentists actually assess and correct real smile problems?

To answer this question, let's turn to the actual smile problems people experience and the general range of solutions available. What you're about to read could be eye-opening for you if you are one of the many who think that their smile problem has no solution – or that every solution is difficult and expensive.

Gummy Smile

Everyone is different. Their muscles work differently. The way they exert them differs in rhythm, force, and duration. Even people of similar body type and weight and strength and bone structure can have widely different ways and speeds of smiling. Another way to put this is to say that the movements of their smiles vary in animation.

People with excess gum may have a static smile and therefore show very little gum. Static smilers, once their smiles are fully operational, show perhaps 0 to 1 mm of gum. However, that same amount of gumminess in an individual who has a dynamic, animated smile will be problematic.

Some dynamic smilers who have a gummy problem will not in fact show it in their basic smile. However, because their muscular movement is animated, they may go too quickly from showing very little tooth and gum in that basic smile to showing a remarkable amount in a large, expanded smile. That sudden display is shocking for people to see. It would be better to show gum all the time than to go from showing a little gum to a lot of gum.

If your smile is animated in this way, the question is whether you show gum nearly all the time or very little until you smile and then, *boom*, it hits everyone in sight.

> *People with dynamic smiles can show more gum.*

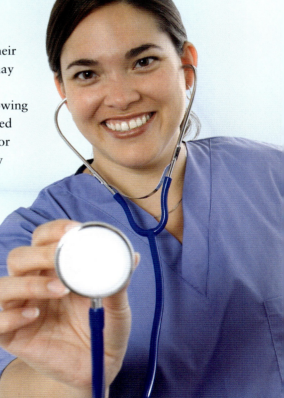

People underestimate the extent to which the shape of the gums affects the shape of the teeth.

Before exploring an aesthetic solution, you and your dentist should determine whether the problem is health-related. If, for instance, you have gingivitis or periodontal disease, that must be dealt with first (and may require the services of a periodontist). This treatment may actually clear up your problem. If not, there are several aesthetic solutions.

Solutions: Gummy smiles can generally be treated either by putting crowns or veneers on the teeth to lengthen them or through a simple correction of the gums. There are five main types of gum solutions.

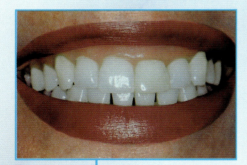

Level 1

Level 1: Sometimes a person will have a gum line that, from birth, has never receded properly. The person appears to have a gummy smile because there is excess gum for the amount of anatomical tooth beneath the gum. X-rays would show the parts of the teeth below the gum that could be exposed.

The excess gum can be easily removed with a procedure no more complicated than removing excess cuticle from your fingernails – though in this case it is done with a laser. The procedure is painless. It doesn't require sutures. A topical anesthetic can be used to make the patient more comfortable. Within five to ten minutes, the excess gum is trimmed away, never to grow again, exposing the long, full, beautiful teeth that have been buried under tissue.

Level 2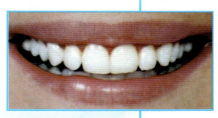

Level 2: Sometimes the teeth are in their correct position in relation to the gums, but too much gum is showing between the teeth and the lip line because the person has a very animated smile.

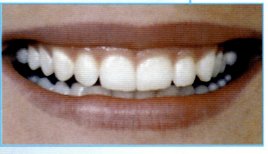

This can be corrected, but it may require a more advanced appraisal to determine how much gum can be removed. This appraisal is done through a procedure called sounding. Using a thin metal probe, the dentist is able to determine how much gum can be removed by the laser without weakening the underlying structure.

Level 3

Level 3: Sometimes gum reduction is clearly needed aesthetically but is problematic dentally because the underlying bone is too close to the gum. Not only does the gum have to be removed, but part of the underlying bone has to be removed as well.

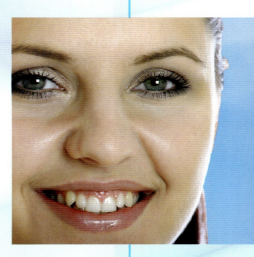

The procedure for doing this usually requires a periodontal and laser treatment. An extended period of time must be allowed for healing before veneers or crowns are placed on the teeth.

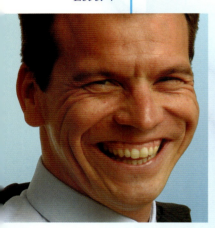

Level 4

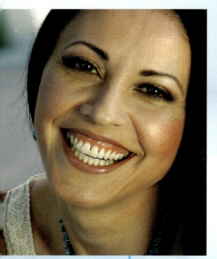

Level 5

Level 4: Some patients clearly have a gummy smile but the teeth, gums, and bone are perfectly positioned, leaving no room to adjust any variable. In such a case, a surgical technique can be performed in which the jaw itself is moved up so that when the patient smiles the gum will not be seen to as great an extent. The gums, bone, and teeth are moved in conjunction with each other to eliminate the gummy smile. This surgical procedure is called a palatal impaction or a Le Forte procedure.

Level 5: There are cases in which the patient's teeth, gums, and bone are in proper aesthetic relationship to each other, but the patient animates too much when smiling – their lip is stretchy, jumping really high and showing too much gum.

The solution here does not involve moving the gums, or the bone, or the teeth – or even performing jaw surgery. It is to do a lip reduction. The patient's lip is actually sutured down so it does not pop up so high during smiling. This procedure is often referred to as Kamer's technique, which effectively lowers the height of the gingival labial synechia. This surgically created synechia partially tethers the upper lip.

One last point here – about the opposite of a gummy smile. Most people are aware of the possibility of removing excess gum. What they don't realize, however, is that gum can actually be added when there is not enough of it. Skin is skin. Skin can be taken from your foot or thigh and put on your back and it will take. The same is true of gum. Gum can be taken from one part of your mouth and grafted or stitched onto another part.

In aged smiles, the teeth have grown worn or discolored.

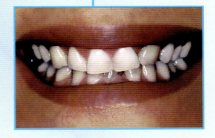

Aged Smile

This is probably the most frequent problem reported by patients. They often complain that their teeth no longer have the appearance they did when they were younger – that they seem to be worn and discolored. They want their teeth revitalized to give their smile a more youthful appearance.

Solution: Just as people can get a more youthful appearance by having plastic surgeon give them a facelift, so they can get a more youthful smile by having a dentist give them a smile lift. The dentist will add length to their worn teeth with crowns, veneers, or bonding, thus recovering the curved smile of the patient's youth. The color of the teeth can easily be changed to a more natural, whiter look.

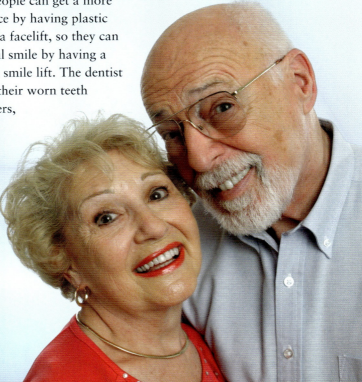

Smile lifts usually involve, at a minimum, the social six – the maxillary anterior teeth – but can in fact involve all of the upper teeth or even all of the teeth.

Inverted Smile

This, after the aged smile, is the second most common smile problem. The cause of the problem is not easily identified by the patient. The problem may not be the result of the aging of the smile. The teeth may in fact not be worn but, for various reasons, have either shifted or drifted, causing the smiles in question to go down, rather than up, at the corners.

The problem is that their upper molars are longer than their front teeth. In a normal smile, the upper lip lifts, creating convexity. In the case of people with inverted smiles, the silhouette of their smile is inverted.

Solution: The mission here is to revert the smile. This is done by various combinations of shortening the upper molars, lengthening the other upper teeth, and building up the lower molars, using crowns or veneers to support the bite change.

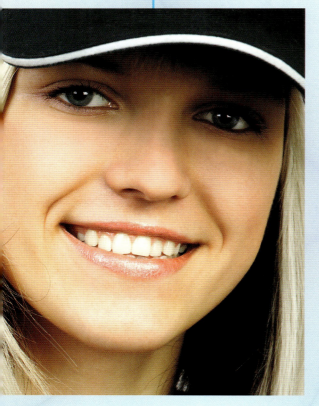

Smiles at times can be as inverted as her hat rim.

Gaps, Crowded, Crooked, Missing

These four problems are typically treated with orthodontic movements but can be treated alternatively with various restorative dental techniques. When the latter approach is chosen, the procedures involved are referred to as "non-orthodontic alignment." Under this category, patients – whether because of age or personal preference – have decided to undergo dental solutions. Unlike orthodontic treatments, the roots are kept in their current position and the teeth are covered with porcelain.

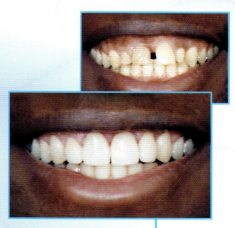

Large spaces between teeth can be considered unattractive.

Following are some general comments on all four of these problems.

Gaps. Most people do not find gaps between teeth attractive overall. The gaps create a dark silhouette, an artificial border, which causes the eye to see black. This bothers us because we are aesthetically trained to want to see continuity in the teeth as they stretch back into the mouth.

This effect is even worse when the teeth are also crooked. Such teeth create curved lines, forming a silhouette that looks like the opposite of an hourglass. The shape of the black against the white creates an odd-looking space that isn't symmetrical to the general look of the teeth. The spaces suggest to our eye an imbalance in form and therefore a lack of genetic harmony – because in such a case the gene that dictates the size of the teeth is out of sync with the gene that dictates the size of the jaw.

The Fix Is In   97

Genetically, then, properly spaced teeth give a signal of good genes overall.

However, even where the teeth are straight, any gaps between them will look unpleasant to most people. One theory is that this look reminds us of our evolutionary past. Early man's lower teeth were much larger than his upper teeth, for the purposes of fighting, hunting, and chewing. However, these larger lower teeth needed spaces to fit into, much as gears need spaces in order to mesh together. This setup was no longer necessary or desired as man evolved and began to eat cooked and softer meats and to use weapons.

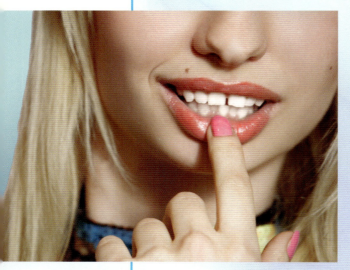

The midline diastema is open to interpretation.

The space between the two front teeth is called the "midline diastema," and it is sometimes thought, by wearers and viewers, to be attractive. Think of the famous actors Madonna, Laura Hutton, and Eddie Murphy. However, there are in fact mathematical and scientific principles for measuring the relative width and proportion of teeth, leading to a more precise determination of what the "perfect gap" should be.

Solution: The following focuses on closing the gap between the two front teeth, but the principles apply to any gaps.

Before a patient and dentist decide to close the midline diastema, the most common gap problem, they should consider five general principles:

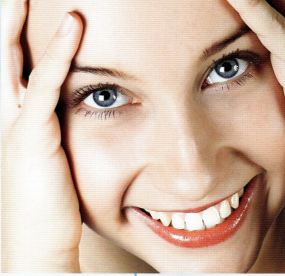

1. The gap may be acceptable – it conforms to the correct proportions of the teeth.
2. The patient may prefer the gap and choose to leave it.
3. The patient may not be prepared to undergo the other treatments that may be necessary to treat and close the gap.
4. The patient may have unreal expectations regarding what they will look like with the gap closed.
5. The closing of the gap may make the other teeth around it look unnatural because of discrepancies in jaw size and tooth size.

If the patient does choose to have the gap closed, the biggest challenge will be adding width to the teeth. If the patient already has teeth that are too narrow, then closing the gap is an opportunity to widen them and give them proper proportion. But more often than not, the teeth are already naturally proportioned. Widening them in order to close the gap creates an unreal and disproportionate appearance. Treating this requires a compensatory process involving one of four variables:

Fixing gaps is all about the overall proportions and what the patient actually wants.

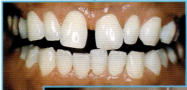

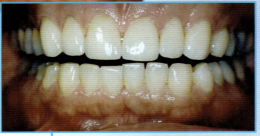

There are several ways to approach gap problems.

1. Gingival height can be increased. By doing this, the dentist is adding length to compensate for the greater width.

2. Incisal length can be increased. Doing this helps achieve proportionality, especially in patients who already don't show enough of their teeth when they smile or speak.

3. The mesial contact (toward the center of the body) or distal contact (toward the outside of the body) can be relocated. When a gap needs to be closed, it is these surfaces that need to be changed. By definition, closing the gap involves two teeth. In deciding how to close the gap, the question must be answered: Do we add to the surface of one tooth or the other tooth, or do we split the difference and add to both?

4. A multidimensional approach is sometimes required. In these cases, many techniques are involved to give natural-looking results. To properly close the gap and create a very natural look, the gum line may have to be reduced; the gingival height increased; incisal length increased; and the teeth built up on either side of the space, thereby minimizing the amount of change that is called for. This technique of spreading the artificial

amounts over many different surfaces so that no one surface involves too much of a change is known as "mortgaging."

Crowded Teeth. Aesthetically, a tooth on its own may be properly proportioned but be perceived as architecturally off because of its twisted and crowded position relative to its adjacent teeth. The way to solve this problem is not that different from what orthodontists would do: creating space and using crowns. At the end of the day, both types of procedures face the same challenge: there are too many teeth overall to fit the arch of the mouth. Space has to be created.

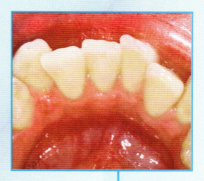

Crowded teeth require careful consideration.

There are two ways to do so. One is to size the teeth down. If the teeth are too wide proportionately for the space they are in, new crowns that are narrower than the original teeth can be fitted into the jaw. In extreme situations a tooth may be so crowded and out of alignment that it may actually have to be extracted, leaving a small space between the adjacent teeth. Part of this approach may involve taking out one or two teeth to create more room. The teeth beside the missing tooth may then be bonded or veneered to give the general appearance of being straight.

The second way is through veneering or adding crowns, to place the teeth into a position relatively forward from where they are – much as orthodontists would do. As the teeth are placed forward, the arch of the mouth is expanded. In this way, the teeth can be given the appearance of being straight.

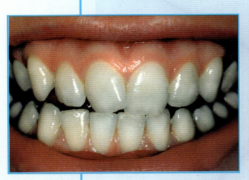

Individual teeth can be crooked or twisted on their own.

Crooked Teeth. This problem is often believed to be the same as that of crowded teeth. The solutions for both are in fact generally the same. However, we often find, in a non-crowded situation, that individual teeth can be crooked or twisted on their own and not as part of a general space problem requiring a complete dentition solution.

It is often possible, when individual teeth are crooked in this way, to realign them with a porcelain veneer or crown. Generally, the tooth must be sanded back on any sides that are out of alignment as a result of the twisting. If the space required to untwist the tooth is wider than what currently exists, it is often possible to sand back a slight amount from each of the adjacent teeth to create the space necessary for the untwisted tooth. If the tooth is in fact greatly twisted, the amount of sanding needed for this realignment may often encroach on the nerve of the tooth, requiring endodontic treatment. This treatment for untwisting teeth is always a calculated risk.

Missing Teeth. There are various ways to replace teeth, depending on the number of teeth missing, the location of the adjacent teeth, the relative root strength of the remaining teeth, the position of the gum line and bony support, and, obviously, cost, time, and individual expectations.

Although removable appliances in the form of acrylic dentures or cast partial dentures are usually more affordable, they are generally not the preferred aesthetic solution.

Removable appliances in general are awkward and inconvenient to wear in the long term.

Bridge work is the most common solution, when clinically possible. However, what is usually required is the crowning of the adjacent teeth to the space. In most cases the patient's teeth accommodate the artificial tooth. However, the fact that it is physically adjacent to the other teeth can cause a bulky and "full" feeling.

Currently, because of their high degree of success, today's innovative new approaches to implant therapy are the preferred route. Placed ideally and properly restored, implants maintain integrity and the natural form to idealize the missing tooth problem.

There are various ways to replace missing teeth.

Bite Problems

There are five main bite problems that relate to smile problems: buck teeth, a prognathic bite, a collapsed bite, a narrow palate, and abfraction.

Buck teeth: In this bite problem, the top front teeth stick out too far. Dentists call this a class 2 occlusion. They solve this problem by grinding away the excess tooth and positioning crowns or veneers over the teeth to move them back to a straighter, more flush alignment with the lip.

Buck teeth

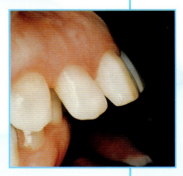

Prognathic bite

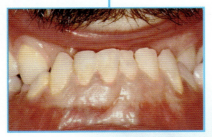

Prognathic Bite: In this condition, the lower jaw sticks out too far. Dentists call this a class 3 bite. It can be solved by essentially veneering the lower teeth backward. Most often, both upper and lower teeth are veneered or crowned and thereby the upper teeth are moved forward, complementing the lower jaw and giving the appearance of properly positioned upper and lower jaws.

Collapsed bite

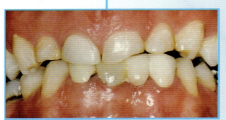

Collapsed Bite: In this condition the teeth, over the years, have worn down and essentially into each other. This decreases the distance between the tip of the nose and chin, which creates an aged look. The teeth are generally too short and appear worn. They are susceptible to fractures. By crowning, bridging, or veneering the teeth, the dentist can restore the height of the patient's bite, increasing the vertical dimension to give the patient a more youthful appearance.

Before: narrow palate

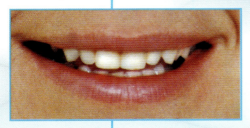

Narrow Palate: People with a narrow palate generally show their front teeth only, giving them a rather rabbity look. The palate may be vaulted as well, in which case an orthdontic appliance can be used to expand the arch. As an alternative, the back teeth can be crowned or veneered and built out to create a fuller arch for the teeth to fit into, thereby establishing a pleasing smile.

Abfraction: Some people notice wedge-shaped areas at their gum line where their fingernail or toothbrush can fit. At these spots the tooth seems to be worn out at the gum line. They often assume, or are told by their dentist, that this is the result of brushing too hard. But in fact it is usually the result of trauma caused by the way they bite down on their teeth. It is a mechanical problem in terms of how the teeth are hitting each other. The pounding of the teeth sends pressure down on the tooth, causing a problem at the weakest point, where the enamel is thinnest. The solution is to bond, veneer, or place crowns on the edges of the teeth, reestablishing a proper bite.

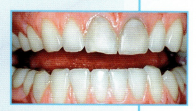
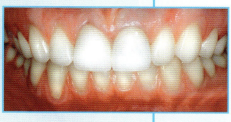

Abfraction before and after

Short Teeth

The amount of tooth showing while talking or smiling is called incisal display. Sometimes a person's top teeth look too short. Dentists can assess this situation by having the patient hold the sound "E" for an extended time to see how much of the front teeth show. Generally the amount should be 2 to 3 mm. If less than that shows, it is either because of unusual wear and tear or because the teeth have not grown in normally.

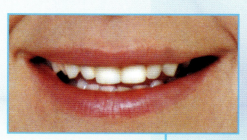

Before: These top front teeth are too short.

The Fix Is In 105

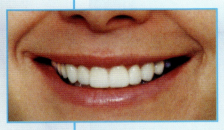

After: Teeth can be lengthened.

Solution: The teeth can be lengthened by bonding, veering, or adding crowns. As was discussed regarding gaps, teeth can effectively be lengthened – by reducing the gum (gingevectomy), especially for patients who have a high lip and show too much of their upper gums when smiling.

Juvenile Smile

Teeth that are short from birth may have the appearance of what dentists call "juvenile smile."

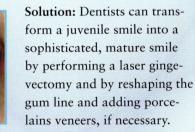

A juvenile smile, before and after veneers and gum surgery.

Solution: Dentists can transform a juvenile smile into a sophisticated, mature smile by performing a laser gingevectomy and by reshaping the gum line and adding porcelains veneers, if necessary.

Skeletal Occlusion

Despite the many different solutions addressed in this chapter to camouflage or otherwise deal with problems by using crowns and veneers, the discrepancy between the teeth and the jaws is sometimes so great, called skeletal occlusion, that there is no other solution but to perform jaw surgery. Either one or both jaws must be moved backward or forward to create a pleasing smile.

Skeletal occlusion

Miscommunication

Let's close this chapter by talking about two situations in which miscommunication is rampant between dentists and patients when it comes to fixing smiles.

"Perfect and Natural"

Patients often ask for something that is actually contradictory, if not oxymoronic. They say, "Give me a perfect, beautiful, Hollywood type of smile that is natural." The dentist is with them – up to that last part about being natural. The problem is that no matter what a dentist does, the porcelain – however real it looks – is not natural. Get over it.

However, in my experience, this request can in fact be met by reaching a certain combination of perfect and imperfect. This requires adhering as much as possible to natural dental anatomy, which at times may be imperfect. The teeth that are made by the ceramist have to have a very natural look by being polychromatic – that is, having not one color but many colors, built and layered into the porcelain. Now here's the trick: There should be some degree of imperfection built into what is created.

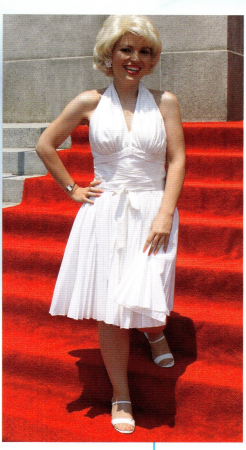

How natural is natural?

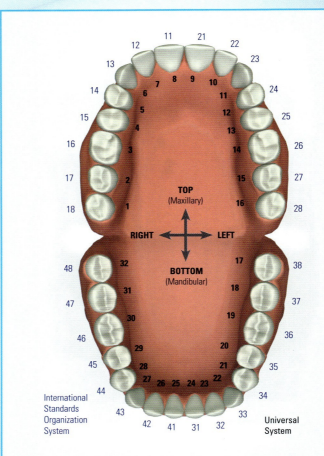

International Standards Organization System

Regardless of which procedures dentists perform in helping patients find their perfect smile, and regardless of which materials they use, whether crowns, veneers, bridges, implants, or others, they will refer to individual teeth by number. Shown here are the two most commonly used numbering systems, the International Standards Organization System (used by Canadian dentists) and the Universal System (used by US dentists).

In other words, while following scientific principles, the ceramist can introduce an artistic element. In this way some sort of harmony between "perfect" and "natural" can be created.

The Neglect of Teens

I have always been baffled by the fact that parents who are so dedicated to helping their children get the best start in life, physically, mentally, and psychologically, nevertheless let them suffer through their teen years with easily fixable dental problems. These parents say, "We'll get them braces when they're kids, but they should wait for aesthetic dentistry until they've finished growing."

But why should these children suffer from a poor image because of dental problems when there is no medical or dental reason not to have the problems fixed? Whitening, bonding, veneering, and so on can be performed on teens as long as all the information is collected and proper consent rules are followed.

I hope this book will encourage parents and children to take a more serious look at aesthetic problems and solutions for teens.

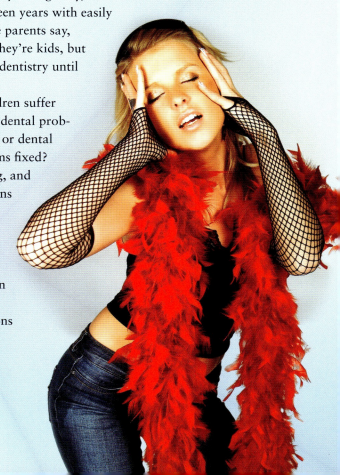

smileline #6

THE ETHICS OF NOSE JOBS AND SMILE JOBS

who?
what?
when?
where?
why?

DECISIONS

Back when cosmetic dentistry was just starting to come on strong, I published an article in a major newspaper commenting on the public misperception of this branch of the profession as aggressively trying to get the public to accept new procedures. I, of course, defended what we were doing as being an acceptable extension and enhancement of dental care.

An editor from that newspaper came to interview me about what I said in the article.

"Don't you think that the sorts of things you talked about in that article are strictly a way for dentists to increase their income?" she asked.

"I beg your pardon?" I said.

"Well, dental income is decreasing, because of fluoride treatments and fewer cavities. Aren't dentists using cosmetic dentistry simply as a gold mine?"

I was offended. "Are you saying that the dentist you trusted five minutes ago to fill a cavity is now going to pick up a drill and file your teeth, simply because they feel they need more work? That all of a sudden they have thrown their ethics out the window?"

We fell into a philosophical discussion about who was responsible for a patient's dental health, the patient or the dentist. I told her that cosmetic dentistry involved providing information about various procedures to patients, who, at the end of the day, were the ones who decided whether they would have the procedures.

I also pointed out that, on her reasoning, no one should ever go to a plastic surgeon for a nose job. If the nose was actually functioning okay, why fix it? The ethics of cosmetic dental surgery were exactly the same, I argued. If it's not immoral to fix a nose, why would it be immoral to fix a crooked smile?

smileline #6

After unburdening myself of these views, I began to sense that the fix was in. Sure enough, she asked me in a teasing tone if I would perform a consultation on her. I sensed that she wanted me to suggest a treatment that she could criticize in her paper. She was quite insistent. "Analyze my smile," she kept saying.

I quickly informed her that she wasn't my patient, and I had no right to comment. "If you want to make an appointment, you should feel free to do so."

After all this, I was expecting a negative article. To my surprise, it was well written and fair. She did explain her initial point of view and concerns but also indicated that in the end it was up to patients to decide what procedures they underwent.

P.S. Months later she did come in for a consultation and had a fair bit of cosmetic dentistry done.

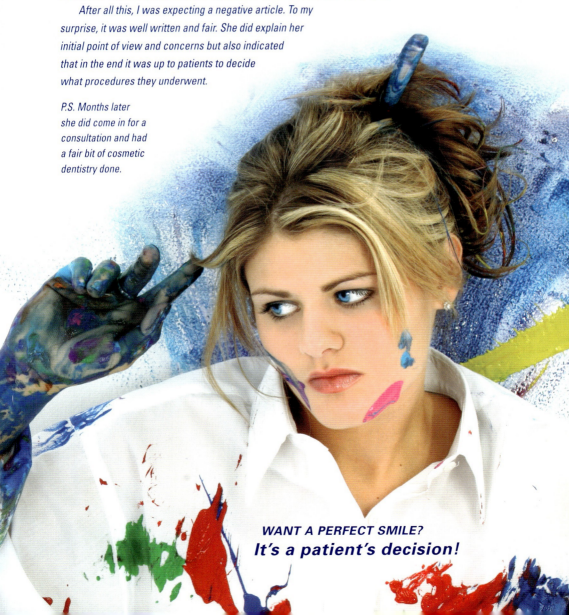

**WANT A PERFECT SMILE?
It's a patient's decision!**

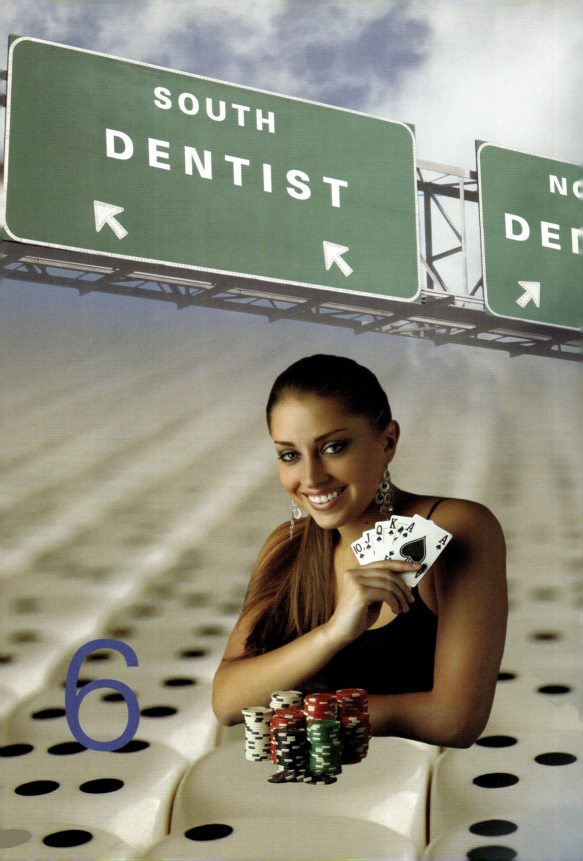

The Consultation Process

Getting Comfortable with Your Dentist and Direction

COSMETIC DENTISTRY HAS THE POWER TO CHANGE YOUR LIFE. It can also be a very serious investment. You need to feel comfortable with the decisions you're making, every step of the way.

During the consultation process, which is the first step toward your new smile, make sure you learn enough about the dentist to be comfortable with their technical skills, personality, and approach. Talking to a dentist will help you understand your treatment options and decide if this is the right dentist for you. You'll probably want to talk to more than one practitioner in order to learn more about your various options. Get a second (or third) opinion – that way you will feel more confident about your choices.

Finding the Right Dentist

Analyze the dentist's portfolio of cases carefully. Make sure that the photos you're being shown are of cases the dentist has actually performed. Sometimes the photos in a dentist's office are of people who haven't had any cosmetic dental work – they simply have great smiles.

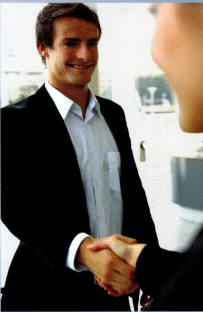

Meet with a few different dentists before you decide.

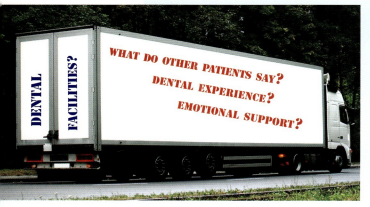

Ask as many questions as you can before you jump on board.

Ask questions based on the treatment plan being proposed to you. Quantity and quality of experience are both important. It's quite all right to say: "I'd like to see other cases that are somewhat similar. How many other cases like mine have you worked on?" Determine whether you're pleased with what you see of the results.

Check references and ask for permission to actually speak to some of the dentist's other patients. Don't forget to look the dentist up on the Internet. What's their educational background? Ask them for their résumé if you haven't been shown one.

What are the dentist's facilities like? Does the clinic seem clean, inviting, comfortable, professional? Does the technical equipment have duct tape holding parts of it together? (It happens.) All of these details will give you clues to the dentist's qualifications.

Does the dentist have a special interest in the kind of work you need or want? Is the practice clearly geared toward this work?

Remember, the dentist is trained to deliver clinical excellence, knowledge, and quality. But these procedures require a strong support team to help make the experience a success. Dentists are generally not able to provide the emotional support necessary on their own. Make sure you have properly assessed the dental team as well as the dentist.

Here's an inside tip: Talk to members of the dentist's support team. If they are familiar with and knowledgeable about the procedure you are contemplating, you can feel confident about the dentist's skill and experience.

If you are considering improving your smile, it's possible that you'll want to consider talking not just to a cosmetic dentist, but also to a plastic surgeon. Depending on your situation, you may need one or the other or you may need both. It makes sense to communicate to everyone on the team. It's similar to renovating a home. You wouldn't undertake serious work without a master plan. The wall paint depends on the plaster work, which must wait for the electrician – who probably needs to synchronize their efforts with the plumbers, and so on.

The critical point is that both the dentist and the

Play your cards carefully as you consider improving your smile.

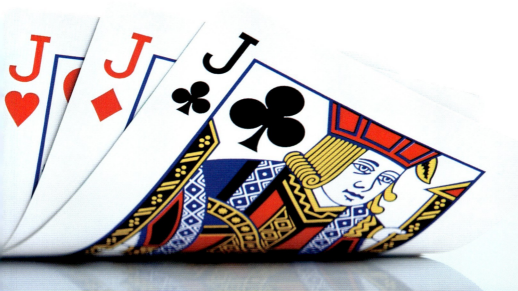

plastic surgeon must take the other's work into account when planning your treatment program. It's very important that every member of the team has the same information at the same time.

Why is this important? Well, here's one example. Let's say you asked your dentist to move your teeth back. This could dramatically change the appearance of your nose – it may now look rather prominent. This kind of problem can be avoided simply by making sure the dentist and plastic surgeon are working on the same page – or, rather, on the same face.

Dentists bring different styles to the way they work.

Communicating with Your Dentist

You're looking for more than just technical skills. You're looking for the right kind of relationship. It would be nice if every dentist could see into your mind and become the dentist you want them to be, but every practitioner is different. Each one brings a certain personality and style to the way they work.

The first step, then, is to look inside yourself for the way you make decisions and work with professionals. For example, consider the issue of control. Imagine that you're buying a formal suit or dress. There are three different basic approaches you may take. You may:

- Look for someone to make the decision for you. ("I have such-and-such an event to go to. What should I wear?")

- Insist on making all of your own decisions. ("Show me what you've got. I'll decide what I want.")
- Operate somewhere between these two extremes. ("Teach me what I need to know, and I'll make an educated decision.")

Communication is paramount. Some dentists are good at saying, "I know what's right for you" and then delivering on it. But if the results are not what you wanted, you may have a problem.

Likewise, other dentists may tell you, "You'd better tell me what you want, because in the end it's *your* mouth." However, you're not a dentist. No matter how much research you've done, you're probably not in a position to know all the issues and technicalities.

It's in your best interest to be as clear and forthcoming as possible about your expectations. It's in your dentist's best interest, meanwhile, to understand the limitations of your knowledge and guide you when necessary. The bottom line is, if you don't end up with the smile you were hoping for, neither of you is going to be happy.

Your best bet is to find a dentist you can relate to easily. The best choice of a dentist for the aesthetic work you desire is one who can take your subjective observations and concerns and explain them to you in objective, scientific terms, as outlined in this book, and then deliver on these insights through skilled treatment.

Keep your eye on the ball to make sure you end up with a smile you're happy with.

Collaborating on Your Treatment Program

The consultation process should involve a detailed analysis of your smile. This will involve the following:

- History and examination
- X-rays
- Determination of your smile pattern: commissure, cuspid, or complex (see chapter two). You have to make sure you're getting a smile that fits your particular pattern, so that the lines follow each other and the effect is natural.
- Photographs. I can't emphasize enough the importance, during the consultation, of a detailed analysis of photographs of your smile. It is vital for your dentist to take into account your smile pattern and the precise stages of your smile.

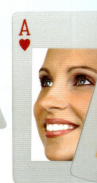

There's nothing more tragic than a patient who, for example, tells their dentist, "I don't show enough teeth when I talk," only to find out, after having their teeth made longer, that they now show far too much tooth when they smile broadly.

- Wax mock-ups to see what your teeth are going to look like. Digital imaging is sometimes done, but this can be highly inaccurate and misleading. Base your decision on digital imaging only if you have been assured that what you're seeing is what you're really going to get as a result of your procedure.

    Always remember that when you're looking at a mock-up of your finished smile, *you're looking at your smile without lips*. The apparent arrangement of the teeth and gums may not tell you how your lips will interact over them. When you talk, for example, your mouth could look too "toothy."

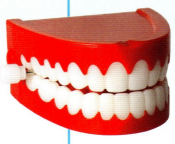

Make sure you have the dentist make a mock-up of your new smile.

Signing a consent form is a worry extinguisher.

- A properly written and executed informed consent contract dealing with the pros and cons of your treatment and potential problems associated with it. This should indicate:
    - How long the work is guaranteed.
    - Whether there will be an extra charge if something goes wrong.
    - What happens if the problem is directly related to the work. What happens if it is indirectly related.

    Consider the following scenario. You have your upper teeth capped, and your dentist guarantees the work for two years. If the cap itself breaks during that time, you get a new cap at no cost. But what if something else occurs as a by-product of the process – say, the tooth

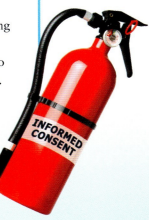

Informed consent forms can go too far (please don't take this one seriously).

Informed Consent

Treatment: Cosmetic Recontouring of Your Chipped Maxillary Central Incisor

You are about to undergo a surgical procedure involving the cutting of a quantity of the enamel from your delicate tooth. In order to ensure that you fully and completely understand the potential risks of this procedure, the following is a thorough review of the possible adverse effects you may encounter in receiving this treatment, from the point at which you arrive at our parking facility.

As you exit your vehicle you may be struck by a car, motorcycle, skateboard, scooter, or other wheeled vehicle, resulting in injuries including but not limited to contusions, abrasions, fractures, concussions, and subdural haematomas. You may trip on gravel, sand, or stones or slip on oil, grease, or brake fluid and impact the pavement causing grave soft tissue and osseous injury. You may be impacted by lightning, falling aircraft, hail, or meteorites, resulting in further serious bodily harm.

Use the elevator at your own risk. Elevators may fall, resulting in isolation for days at a time. Use of the stairs may entail risk of angina, cardiac arrest, or falling to a horribly bloody mangled death.

On entry to the dental clinic, various contagious agents may be inhaled, including influenza virus, staph aureus, strep pyogenes, as well as The Plague, anthrax, and ebola. These may result in serious illness, including huge fungating sores, pus-filled lung masses, flesh-eating disease, or death.

In the operatory the chair will be placed in the supine position. This may result in syncope, ataxia, hyperventilation, and/or paranormal hallucinations.

A course flex disc will be applied with moderate pressure to the traumatic incisal chip site. Vibrations and a noxious odor of burning teeth are common symptoms. A sharp piercing pain resonating through your tooth and jaw may occur as the heat of the procedure builds up a pulpal response.

Complications from this procedure may include but are not limited to swelling; damage to and possible loss of other teeth, fillings, or other dental work; infection or abscess; pain; significant bleeding; sinus or nasal problems; poor healing; loss of bone; fracture of the jaw; injury to nerves which may cause pain, numbness, or tingling of the lips, chin, face, mouth, teeth, and/or damage to the ability to taste; and possible stretching of the corners of the mouth with resultant cracking and bruising.

Finally, although a good cosmetic result is hoped for, it cannot be guaranteed. Have a nice day!

_____   _____   _____
Patient/Guardian Signature   Witness Signature   Date

dies from the capping process and you now need a root canal? You have not paid for a root canal, so it's not going to be covered under your guarantee.

- Discuss exactly who will do what. What work will the dentist do? What parts of the procedure will be performed by other technicians?
- Also go over the kinds of materials that will be used. In particular, find out about the ceramist and their work.

A smile is only as good as the ceramic work that goes into it. Most dentists in North America do not identify the maker and supplier of the ceramic work. In many cases, ceramic work will be contracted to an off-site lab. Meet the ceramist, if possible. That way you can get personal assurance regarding their involvement in the case and commitment to the results.

There are as many types of ceramic material as there are cars, from Chevrolet ceramics all the way to Ferrari ceramics, with price tags to match. Understand what ceramic materials you're paying for, and why. Why has the dentist chosen this material for your particular problem? The materials used can make a huge difference to the end result of your treatment.

When you and your dentist have selected all the right pieces, you're ready to go.

Understand the Range of Your Treatment Options

Is your smile problem isolated, involving only a few teeth, or does it go deeper, involving many teeth or even the overall structure of your bite? The key is to define and understand the problem and the various approaches that may help to correct it.

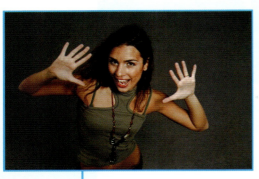

Make sure you count all your options.

For minor tooth problems, you're looking for a minor fix. For major tooth problems, you're looking for a major fix. Certainly it's easier to deal with a specific problem. For example, if you have lost a tooth, then it's easy to live with the space, or get an implant, denture, or bridge. But the greater the problem, the more comprehensive a solution you need. Dentists may not be able to correct the problem of short teeth by simply lengthening the teeth – they may have to work with the gums, or change the overall bite.

It's important to understand that there are several potential treatments for every problem. There may be four different treatment choices for your particular situation, or there may be only two. Just make sure that your dentist explains the full spectrum of treatment options. Ask what your options are, all the way from doing nothing to pursuing the most comprehensive possible course of treatment.

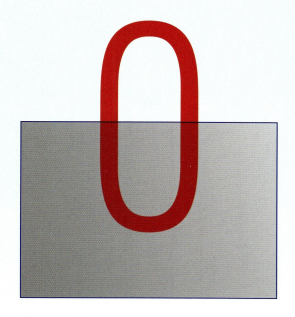
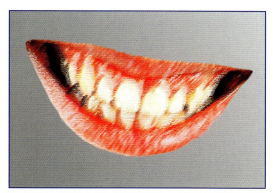
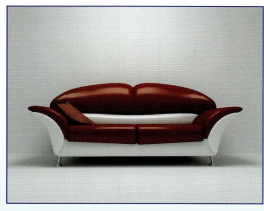

check us out @ www.smilingfurniture.com

THE STORY OF A SMILE TO RE-LIE ON

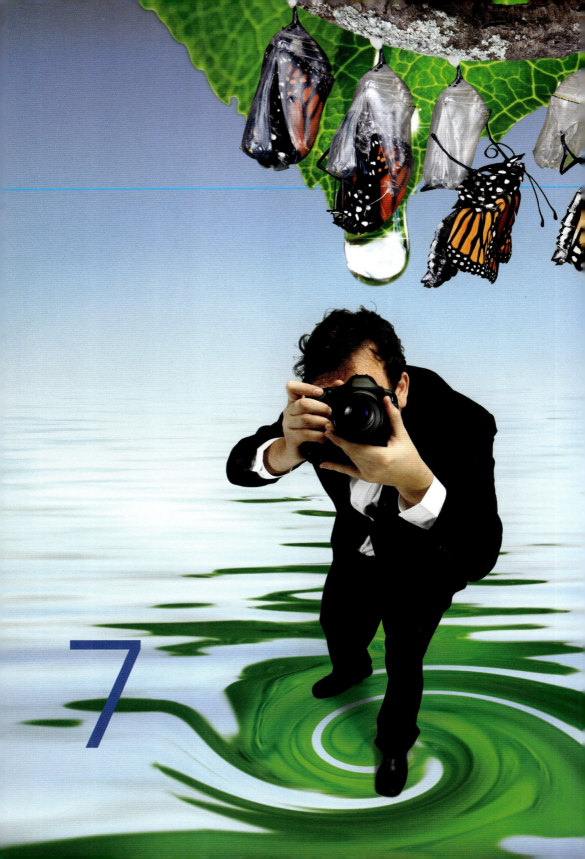

7

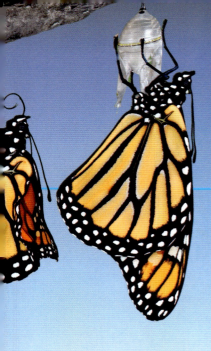

Before and After

A Photo Gallery of Smiles

GIVEN TODAY'S MAKEOVER MANIA, many of us are suspicious of before-and-after images. We assume that photographers, camera operators, and computers have been pressed into service to dazzle our eyes and dull our intellects. I can assure you that no photographic prestidigitation has been employed to enhance the pictures of smiles in this book. I have chosen ones that give a realistic sense of what the average patient can expect. Moving teeth to fit the smile, filling gaps, and whitening can make a dazzling difference. Yet the ultimate benefit is when an outsider does not actually notice the dental work and says, "You look fabulous. Did you change your hairstyle?" We appreciate our patients' trust in allowing us to use the following photos, but in most cases we have altered names and facts to protect their privacy.

Uncovering the beauty within.

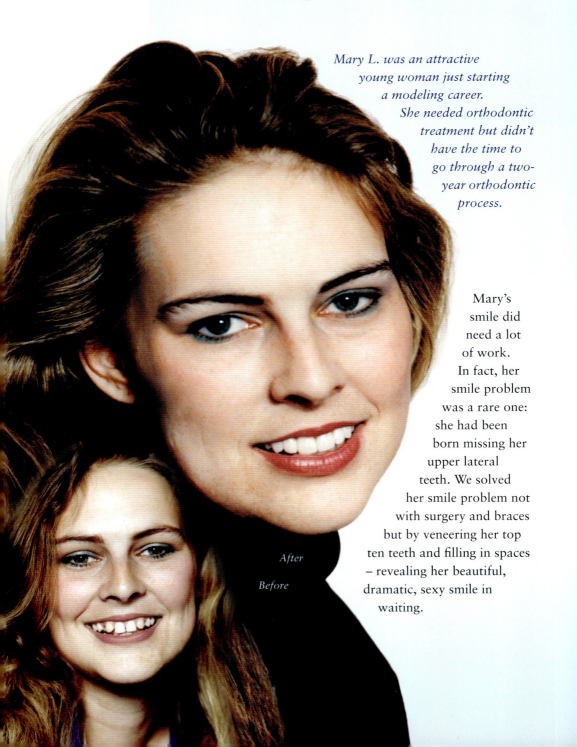

smilegallery #1

Mary L. was an attractive young woman just starting a modeling career. She needed orthodontic treatment but didn't have the time to go through a two-year orthodontic process.

Mary's smile did need a lot of work. In fact, her smile problem was a rare one: she had been born missing her upper lateral teeth. We solved her smile problem not with surgery and braces but by veneering her top ten teeth and filling in spaces – revealing her beautiful, dramatic, sexy smile in waiting.

After

Before

smilegallery #2

Heather K. was in her first year as a teacher and felt that her smile was not going to win her any brownie points with her students.

Heather had been born with very crooked and twisted teeth, and though she was the life of the party and willing to take a risk, her smile had always caused her to feel awkward and self-conscious. We transformed her smile by veneering her top ten teeth, and whitening all of her front teeth, top and bottom.

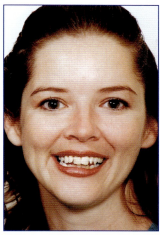

Before

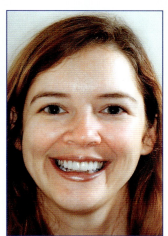

After

smilegallery #3

Singer and song writer Danielle Smith, also known as Fidget, needed a beautiful, sexy smile for her website photo and publicity shots – and her concert performances.

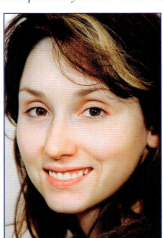

Before

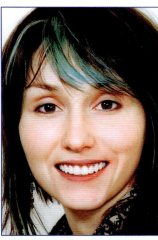

After

Danielle had a great smile to begin with, courtesy of earlier work done by another dentist. But, as she put it, "I've cranked my music up and now I want to crank up my smile." We were pleased to help, by giving her a new set of veneers.

smilegallery #4

Pepe of Bogart's Men Clothing – who had been bringing a smile to my face as my tailor for years – had an unusual assessment of his smile: "I hate it – it looks too Italian."

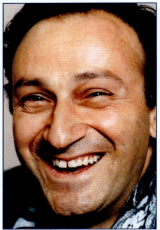

Before

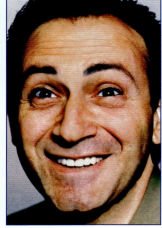

After

I told him I was quite sure there was no such thing as an Italian smile. After I closed the gap between his middle top teeth and dressed his smile up with ten porcelain veneers, I asked him if his smile still looked Italian. "Yes, it does," he said, "but I don't care – I love it."

smilegallery #5

Charlene F., a volleyball player, hated her gummy smile – to the point that she always covered it up, even after a dramatic play on the court.

Charlene was a natural competitor in several sports. She told us that she was after any advantage she could get when performing for juries and fans. We performed gum surgery on her and gave her a new set of porcelain veneers, and she flashed a big smile when she later won a body-building championship.

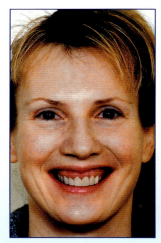

Before

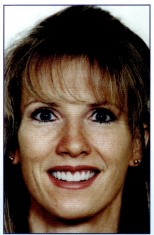

After

smilegallery #6

Everyone knows funny guy Mark Breslin, the standup comic and CEO of Yuk Yuks (and the writer of this book's Afterword).

Mark wasn't worried about stage fright – not his, anyway. He wanted to make sure people were laughing at his jokes and not shielding their eyes from his teeth. We were pleased to contribute to his act by veneering his twelve upper teeth. He told us later that because we didn't let him talk during the whole procedure, we were the toughest crowd he had ever worked.

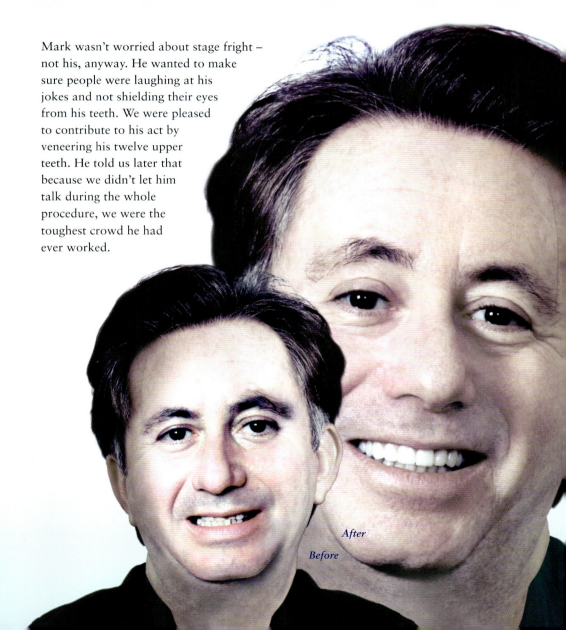

After

Before

smilegallery #7

Jack P., a real estate agent, was the king of leasing office space, but he couldn't get rid of the spaces between his teeth.

Jack was already tremendously successful as a top real-estate salesman. Showing one of the traits that made him a winner, Jack felt an attractive smile would help keep him at the top of his game. We booked him for several sessions and did some mortgaging of our own, veneering most of his teeth to fix their unevenness and gaps. Jack's instincts paid off – he's one agent who's always busy, whether the market is hot or cold.

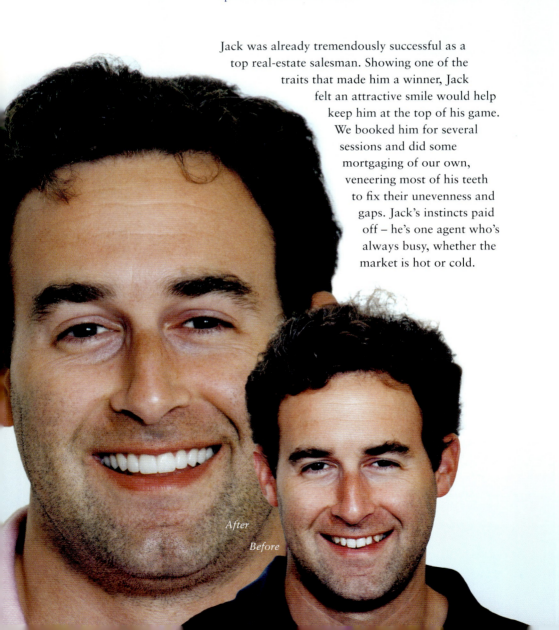

After

Before

smilegallery #8

This quiet woman, Joan S., didn't like what she was told: that she needed extractions and braces to fix her smile.

Joan did have unusually crooked teeth, and her case proved a bit of a challenge. But we were able to give her a great smile by veneering her teeth to give them a more even look. She actually appeared on national TV later to describe her experience in finding her perfect smile.

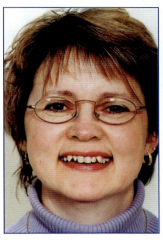

Before

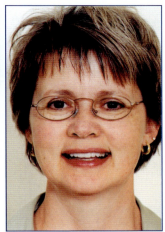

After

smilegallery #9

As if being a teenager was not pressure enough, Tamara F.'s smile was making her feel self-conscious around her peers.

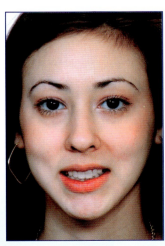

Before

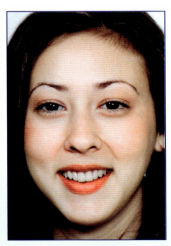

After

Tamara's teeth were nicely shaped but were stained as a result of tetracycline, an antibiotic. We were able to give a boost to her confidence by whitening and veneering her top front six teeth.

smilegallery #10

Alexandra K. was a high-end designer whose beautiful smile was already in fashion. That wasn't good enough for her, however.

Alexandra, who made fabulous leather clothing, told us that she didn't consider her smile good enough – that she wanted a cutting-edge smile to match her cutting-edge designs. We whitened and veneered her front teeth and were pleased when she later told us that she considered her smile tailor-made for her.

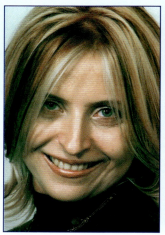

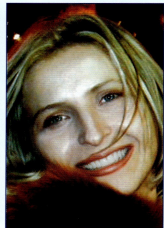

Before   *After*

smilegallery #11

Roberto D., editor of a health magazine, was another patient who started with a good smile.

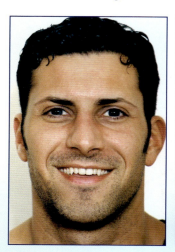

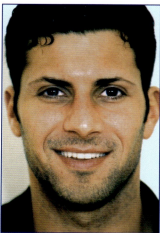

But Roberto knew that he needed help, not with his smile itself, but with something others couldn't see – his bite. He had a gap at the front of his mouth between his top and bottom teeth when he closed his back teeth. We fixed this by using veneers to lengthen his front teeth.

Before   *After*

smilegallery #12

Robyn D. was frustrated when several dentists told her they didn't want to risk making any changes to her smile.

Most people would have ended their mission after just one or two dentists turned them away, but not Robyn. She's a good example of the value of persisting until you are successful in your search for the perfect smile. She was also a good example of how a small and seemingly insignificant adjustment – we veneered her front six teeth – is often all it takes to make a great smile out of a good one.

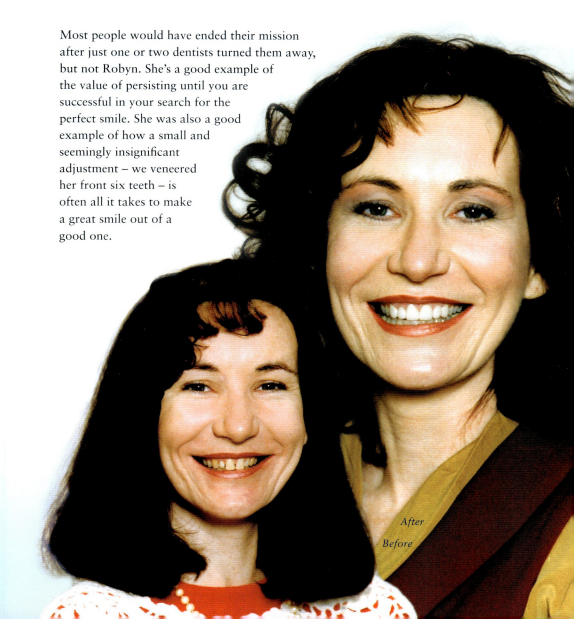

After
Before

The Perfect Smile

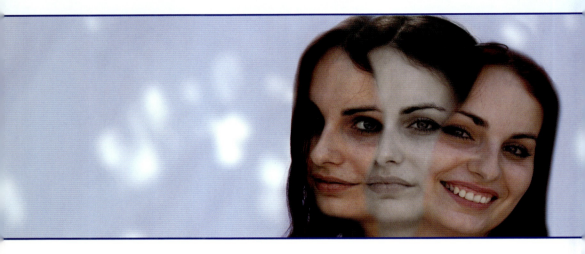

happens in

... but lasts

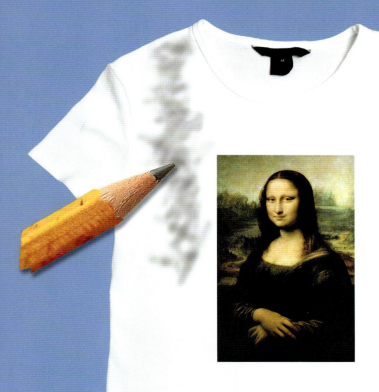

a moment
forever

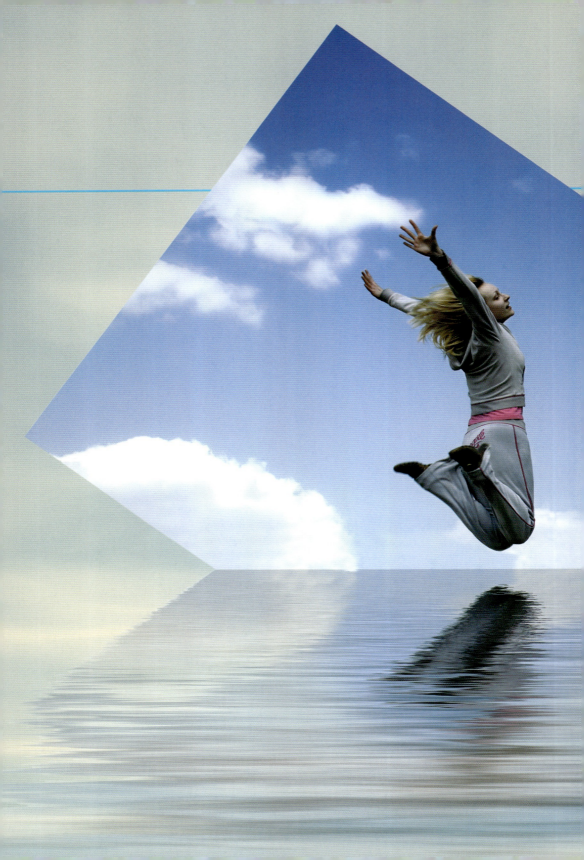

Afterword

"FUN" AND "DENTIST" ARE TWO WORDS RARELY ASSOCIATED WITH EACH OTHER. Usually the word "dentist" suggests words like "pain," "discomfort," and "humorless guy looming over you."

But it doesn't have to be this way. A lot of changes have happened in modern dentistry. When I was a child, my dentist was *reactive* – he took care of some trouble in my mouth. Now, a dentist can be *pro-active* – he can change my smile, and change my life.

OK, but is it *fun*? It can be, with the right attitude. Attitude is everything. You've got to emphasize the positive. So here are some of the things to look forward to on your next trip.

First of all, the dental hygienist is almost always a hot babe. She'd better be. If you spent your days telling strangers to "spit" you'd wind up an old maid if you weren't a hottie to compensate. So enjoy the company of your attractive and sweet-tempered filer and scraper.

Next, the dental waiting room. It now has magazines you might actually want to read. And someone with at least a year of design school picked out some relaxing earth tones and pastels, so you no longer feel you're in a socialist housing project in Malmo, Sweden.

The dentist gives you drugs. This cannot be overemphasized. One new development is "dentistry while asleep." One word of caution, however: this should apply to the patient, not the dentist.

The dental office has been turned into an entertainment multiplex. At my last visit, I had my choice of an iPod, satellite radio, cable TV, video game, and DVD player. When the chair went back, I thought for a moment I was on a first-class flight overseas.

You can even bring your own entertainment. But I suggest a CD of the Dead Kennedys might be counterproductive to the experience, and that only the truly perverse would bring a copy of *Marathon Man* to watch during the procedure.

Next: the dentist. Good news: no longer a nerd!

That's right! The modern dentist now comes with attachments of decent wardrobe, subtle cologne, educated opinions, and witty banter. Of course, you're stuffed with cotton and can't banter back, but what a great opportunity to practice those mime skills!

Fun at the dentist can mean playing practical jokes in and out of the chair. I like to scream my head off during a simple consultation for the benefit of those in the waiting room who look suitably freaked as I then walk out whistling and waving.

Some dentists have added spa treatments to their procedures. At the present this is limited to hand massages and basic reflexology, but give it time and before long, mani/pedis will become standard and visits will be scheduled weekly, instead of biannually.

So instead of approaching your next visit to the dentist with dread, make it a trip full of fun and laughter. Your dentist will be only too happy to reciprocate with sensitivity and wit. Make friends with your dentist. After all, it's not like he's a ... lawyer.

MARK BRESLIN
CEO, Yuk Yuks

I enjoyed the journey.
... Did you?

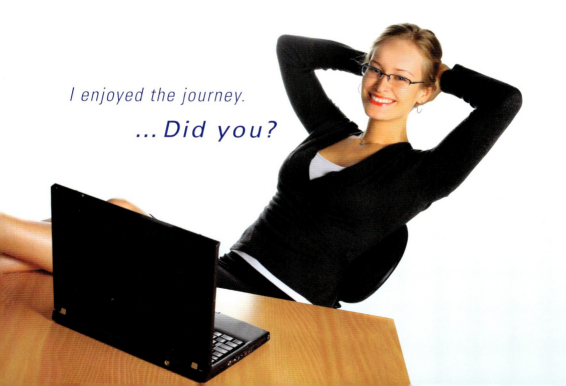

A SMILE TAKES A SECOND
... BUT LASTS FOREVER

Nature's use of the Golden Mean can be found in the animal, vegetable, and mineral kingdoms.

Try looking at a photograph of yourself in profile with your lips closed.

Virtually all of us, whatever our background or education, know beauty when we see it.

Your teeth should be lighter than your skin tone.

DECISIONS

We all smile in the same language.